Rihem Mezrigui
Saoussen Chouchene
Nadia Yacoubi

# Artificial intelligence at the service of hematology

Rihem Mezrigui
Saoussen Chouchene
Nadia Yacoubi

# Artificial intelligence at the service of hematology

## From early diagnosis to personalized treatment

ScienciaScripts

**Imprint**



Cover image: www.ingimage.com

This book is a translation from the original published under ISBN 978-620-6-72279-3.

Publisher:
Sciencia Scripts
is a trademark of
Dodo Books Indian Ocean Ltd. and OmniScriptum S.R.L publishing group

120 High Road, East Finchley, London, N2 9ED, United Kingdom
Str. Armeneasca 28/1, office 1, Chisinau MD-2012, Republic of Moldova, Europe
Printed at: see last page
**ISBN: 978-620-8-12300-0**

## Table of contents

# INTRODUCTION

In the medical field, technological advances have considerably extended the capabilities of automated systems, and hematology is no exception to this trend. Since the beginning of the 19th century, the hematology laboratory has benefited from a series of advances, improving the precision and efficiency of automated diagnostic systems.

The next stage of evolution in hematology will be marked by the integration of artificial intelligence (AI), which is already beginning to transform traditional methods of blood and hematopoietic tissue analysis **[1]**.

These advances promise unparalleled precision in diagnosis, decision-making and choice of therapeutic alternatives in clinical hematology. **[2]**.

However, the basic concepts are often unfamiliar to clinicians and healthcare professionals, and a good understanding of AI techniques is crucial to streamlining its uses and promising precision medicine.

This thesis aims to explore, through an in-depth literature review, the current applications of AI in hematology, assess the opportunities it offers for improving patient care, and identify the challenges associated with its implementation.

We begin by elucidating the foundations and techniques of AI, using specific medical terminology, and then examine its applications in the diagnosis, prognosis and treatment of hematological disorders. Finally, we discuss the prospects of technological advances for tomorrow's medicine, and highlight the challenges and limitations that researchers and practitioners face in using these promising technologies.

# 1. THEORETICAL FOUNDATIONS OF ARTIFICIAL INTELLIGENCE

In the medical sector, AI is playing a crucial role in transforming the way healthcare professionals diagnose, treat and prevent disease. This convergence between IT and medicine has paved the way for a new era of more personalized, efficient and accessible healthcare. In this chapter, we begin with an introduction to the basics of artificial intelligence. We explain the various emerging approaches and methods, drawing on concrete examples of applications in the medical field.

## 1.1. The basics of how artificial intelligence systems work

AI is a vast field that encompasses a set of theories, algorithms and techniques aimed at creating systems capable of emulating human cognitive processes. This is done by using computers to run sophisticated computer programs that process and analyze massive data in a way similar to the way a human brain would. **[2]**.

The foundations of AI rest on an essential synergy between algorithms and massive data, commonly referred to as *"Big Data."* **[3]**. These two elements are interdependent, and form the cornerstone of AI's meteoric rise in many fields of application.

### 1.1.1. Big *Data*

The digitization of various areas of daily life, particularly in the medical field, has generated a voluminous amount of data, both structured and unstructured. To exploit this data, the use of sophisticated, well-structured management tools is essential.

*"Big Data"* therefore refers to extremely large and complex data sets that exceed the capacity of traditional data management and analysis methods **[4]**.

The automated processing of these immense volumes of data, commonly known *as "datamining"*, brings to light subtle correlations between them. By harnessing this massive data, AI algorithms can identify trends, patterns and relationships within medical information, facilitating more informed decision-making by healthcare professionals **[5]**. For example, in medical diagnostics, automated data analysis can help spot early signals of disease, enabling early diagnosis and rapid intervention.

The medical application of *datamining-based* decision support also contributes to the optimization of treatment protocols. By analyzing patients' responses to different therapies, it becomes possible to adjust treatment approaches in a personalized way, thus improving the effectiveness of care **[5]**.

### 1.1.2. Algorithm

An algorithm is an organized, precisely defined set of instructions and operations that enables systems to learn patterns from collected data and make intelligent decisions to accomplish a given task. It relies on input data to generate a specific result in a **finite amount of** time **[6]**. A computational sequence can be seen as a concrete example of an algorithm, where a series of operations is performed sequentially to achieve a desired result.

In the medical field, the process that leads to a diagnosis is also based on an underlying algorithm. The inputs are the patient's medical data, such as symptoms, medical history and test results. This information is then analyzed according to criteria and rules established by medical experts. This analysis ultimately results in a medical diagnosis, which is the output of this algorithm **[5]**.

## 1.2.Fundamental approaches to artificial intelligence

AI is defined as a structure capable of thinking and making decisions. It can automatically perform actions or tasks through a process *called Machine Learning (ML). Deep Learning (DL)*, a more advanced form of *ML*, mimics the functioning of the human brain, enabling AI to analyze, understand, learn and perform tasks based on its interpretations and choices **(Figure 1). [7]**.

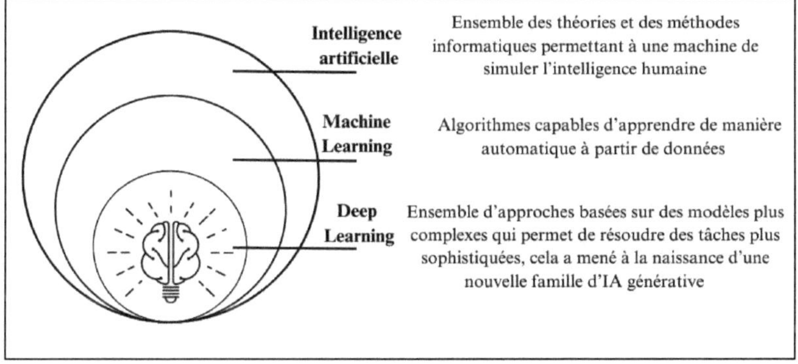


**Figure 1 General diagram of artificial intelligence [7]**

### 1.2.1. Machine learning

#### 1.2.1.1. Definition and uses

Machine learning, also known as ML, is an approach to data analysis that automates the process of creating analytical models. It is the main branch of modern AI, based on the notion that systems can acquire knowledge from data, discern patterns and make decisions with minimal human intervention. Machine learning algorithms can be employed in a variety of fields, such as image and speech recognition, natural language processing, as well as decision-making **[8]**.

#### 1.2.1.2. Differences from traditional programming

ML and traditional programming represent two distinct approaches to computer problem solving. **Table I** presents a detailed comparison of the distinguishing features between ML and traditional programming algorithms, based on Alassadi and ***Ivanauskas*** **[9]**.

**Table ICharacteristic differences between traditional programming and *Machine Learning* [9]**

| Features | Traditional Programming | *Machine Learning* |
|---|---|---|
| **Principle** | Follow explicit logical instruction sequences coded by a programmer | Learning from data, identifying patterns |
| **Strict rules** | Strict rules to anticipate for precise operation | Adjust parameters to optimize performance |
| **Use** | Problems with well-understood rules that are stable over time | Complex problems, evolving or ill-defined rules |
| **Learning** | No learning techniques | Learning from examples and data |
| **Adaptability** | No adaptability | Adaptability to changing and complex situations |
| **Flexibility** | Less flexible, programmed for specific conditions | More flexible, capable of handling complex data |
| **Complexity** | Often simpler to implement | Perhaps more complex, but suitable for complex tasks |

Traditional programming is therefore appropriate for problems with clear, stable rules, while ML excels at solving complex, adaptive problems by learning from the data **(Figure 2) [9]**.

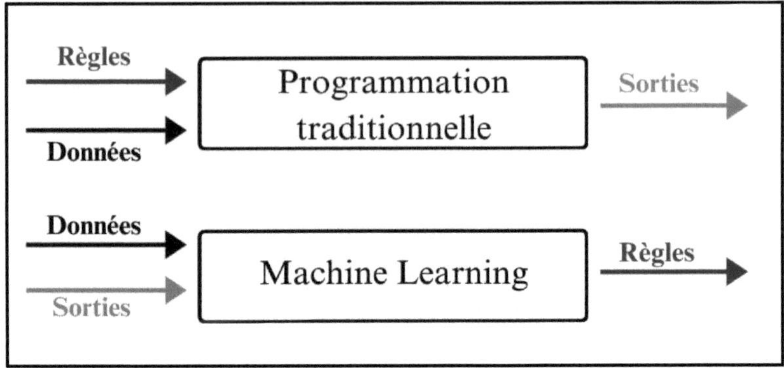


**Figure 2 Diagram illustrating the differences between traditional programming and *Machine Learning*. [9]**

### 1.2.2. Artificial neural networks or *"Deep Learning"*

DL is a subcategory of ML that focuses on using deep artificial neural networks to learn hierarchical representations of data **[8]**. It is a computer processing system strongly inspired by the functioning of the biological nervous system.

An artificial neural network primarily comprises a large number of interconnected computational neurons, called perceptrons, which work in a distributed fashion to collectively interpret input data in order to optimize the final output **[10]**.

Each artificial neuron acts as a basic processor, receiving a variable set of inputs from upstream neurons. Each input is accompanied by a weight *(*w) that expresses the intensity of the connection. Each core processor produces a single output, then branches out to provide signals to a variable number of downstream neurons. Each connection to these neurons is also defined by a specific weight **[11]**. It is thus designed to be a simplified representation of a biological neuron, as shown in **figure 3.**

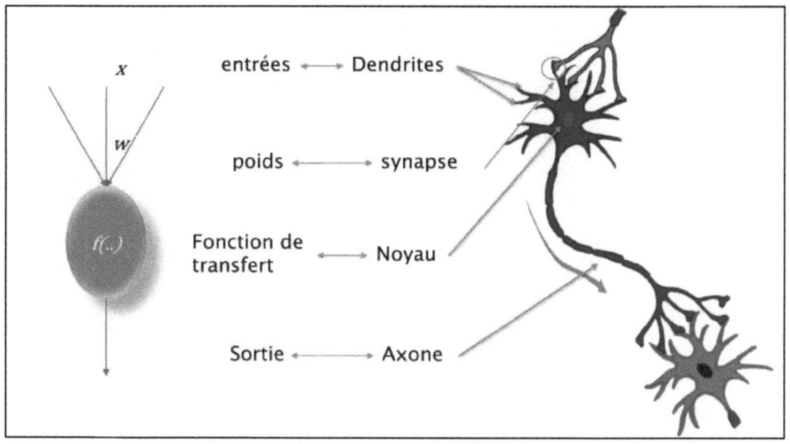


**Figure 3 Analogy between a biological neuron and an artificial neuron artificial neuron (perceptron) [12]**

The dendrites of a biological neuron receive electrochemical signals from other neurons, whereas in a perceptron, the inputs correspond to the dendrites and are weighted by weights. The nucleus of a biological neuron processes the signals received and generates an action potential, whereas in an artificial neuron, the weighted sum of inputs, plus a bias, is subjected to an activation and transfer function to produce the output. The electrochemical signal propagates along the axon of a biological neuron and is transmitted to other neurons via synapses, just as the output of a perceptron is transmitted to other neurons in the network. Synapses, which are connections between axons and dendrites in a biological neuron, enable the transmission of electrochemical signals, while in an artificial neuron, weights associated with inputs play a similar role by modulating the importance of input signals **[11]**.

A single perceptron does not have the ability to accurately approximate any continuous function. In fact, its modeling power is limited. However, it is possible to combine several perceptrons to form a neural network. This leads to the creation of more powerful models known as *"multilayer perceptron"* (MLP ). An MLP consists of an input layer, an output layer and a variable number of intermediate layers called *"hidden layers"*. Each unit is designated by a neuron and linked to all the neurons in the next layer **(Figure 4). [13]**.

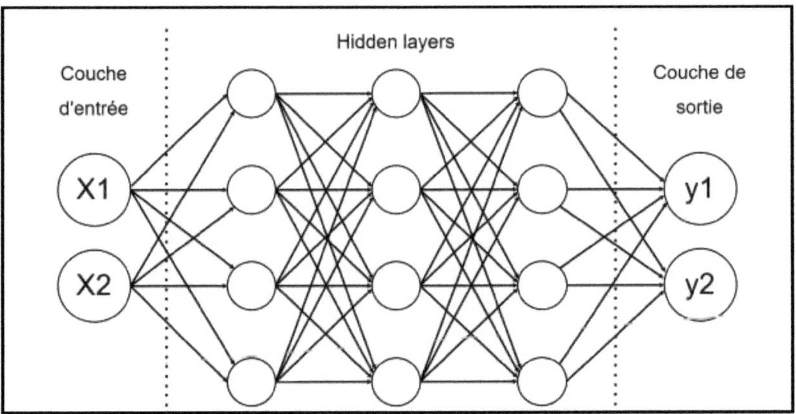


**Figure 4 Schematic diagram *of* a *multilayer perceptron* [13]**

#### 1.2.2.1. Convolutional neural network

A convolutional neural network ( *"Convolutional Neural Network"* or CNN) can be conceptualized as a variant of a traditional artificial neural network, but is distinguished by a specific organization of its neural layers in several dimensions. Unlike a conventional neural network, where each neuron is connected to a neuron in the previous layer, in a CNN, the neurons in a given layer are sporadically interconnected with a restricted subset of neurons in the previous layer. This particular structure enables the CNN to incorporate selective information into its architecture, making it effective for processing complex data, such as images or temporal signals **[14]**.

As layers are added to a CNN, its complexity increases, enabling it to discern more features or areas in an **image [15]**.

Starting with basic features, it develops the ability to perceive more complex attributes, such as object shape and larger-scale elements, until eventually being able to recognize the image as a whole **[16]**. CNNs, known to give excellent results in image recognition tasks, have been extensively researched for their application in the medical field, notably in cell classification, karyotyping automation and radiological interpretation, using an image dataset **[17]**.

#### 1.2.2.2. Recurrent neural network

The recurrent neural networks ( *"Recurrent Neural Networks"* or RNN ) are conventional neural networks with embedded recurrent connections. These additional connections establish links between the hidden layers of the network. They include parameters (weights) **[11]**. Unlike direct-propagation networks, RNNs have a structure that allows information to flow in both directions, as illustrated in **Figure 5**, bringing them closer to biological networks. **[11]**.

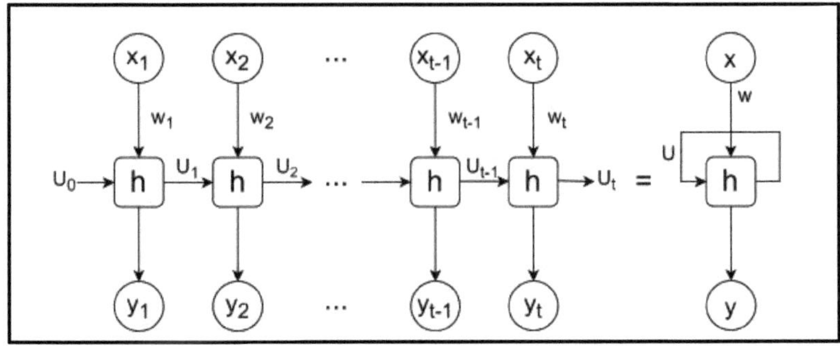


**Figure 5 Prediction scheme for a recurrent neural network t [18]**

This bi-directional capability allows analyzed signals to be influenced by previously received signals, creating an operation similar to a short-term system memory. These networks, especially since they have been improved by *"Long Short Term Memory"* (LSTM) architectures with internal memory cells, are proving particularly suitable for text, sound and video analysis, where the temporal dimension plays a crucial role. **[19]**.

### 1.2.2.3. Internal memory cells

RNNs, designed to handle sequential data such as sequences of words in a sentence or one-off events in a time series, have one limitation: they can look back in time over only about ten time intervals. This means they have difficulty capturing long-term data **[19]**.

This limitation is due to a problem called " *vanishing gradient"* or *"explosive gradient"*. Basically, during training, the gradients (which indicate how to adjust the network weights) become either very small (*"vanishing"*) or very large (*"explosive"*), making learning unstable and difficult **[19]**.

To solve this problem, LSTMs were developed. They are able to store and use information over long sequences of time, making them much more effective for tasks requiring long-term data understanding. What's more, they are based on mechanisms that are biologically plausible. Similar to simple RNN, LSTMs also have a fixed structure, deployed over time, but the repeated unit itself has a different structure. Each unit of an LSTM comprises several different types of modules that interact to confer memory on the model **[19]**. The structure of an LSTM can be seen in **figure 6**.

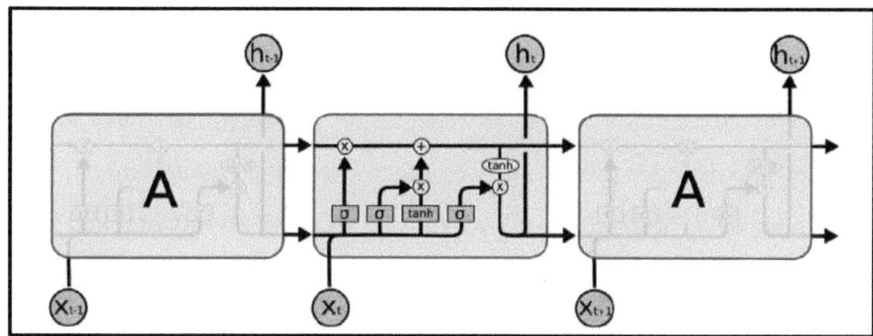

**Figure 6Structure of a *Long Short Term Memory* unit [20]**

Depending on the complexity of the network built (i.e. the number of layers and neurons), LSTMs can learn over much longer sequences of time than traditional RNNs. This makes them very powerful for tasks such as machine translation, speech recognition and many other sequence processing applications. **[19]**.

#### 1.2.2.4. *"Transformer*: neural network

To explore information, human beings typically use their "attention mechanism" to filter out irrelevant information while focusing on the meaningful parts of the data encountered in everyday life. Inspired by this observation **[21]**researchers have designed attention mechanisms for deep learning that filter homogeneous data while paying attention to the most important elements. **[22]**.

This is how the *"Transformer"* was created. This innovative DL model is designed to handle sequences, i.e. ordered sets of elements (such as words in a sentence). It takes a sequence as input and generates predicted probabilities as output. This enables the *"Transformer"* to capture long-term dependencies in the data without needing to depend on the recurrent architecture **[23]**.

It is mainly composed of the attention mechanism and has either an encoder, a decoder or an encoder-decoder structure. The choice of architecture is determined by the nature of the task at hand, which we'll go into in more detail in the following sections.

The encoder generates a vector representation (*"embedding "*) of an input sequence. The decoder produces a sequence from this *embedding*.

The decoder of a "*Transformer"* is made up of successively stacked layers, each taking as input the output of the last encoder. At each decoder stage, this system explores whether crucial information is present in the past, i.e. in the encoder. In terms of analogy, when translating a sentence, this would be equivalent to revisiting the sentence to be translated at each word/step.

Recently, " *Transformers"* have also pollinated the field of medical image analysis, where they are used for disease diagnosis **[22]**.

### 1.3. Techniques and types of task performed by artificial intelligence

ML algorithms are tools capable of solving different types of prediction problems. To make these predictions, the model uses data, also known as instances or observations, and statistics provides a methodological framework for modeling these data. In the case of a data table, each row represents one of these observations. The model then uses these observations to make a prediction **[18]**.

A model's parameters determine how it makes predictions from a given observation, thus defining its behavior **[18].**

ML comprises three key approaches: supervised, unsupervised and reinforcement learning. Supervised learning uses labeled data to train predictive models, while unsupervised learning explores structures in unlabeled data. Reinforcement learning introduces interaction, with the agent adjusting its actions to maximize rewards. Combined, these approaches enable artificial intelligence to solve a wide range of problems, illustrating the versatility of the field **(Figure 7) [2]**.

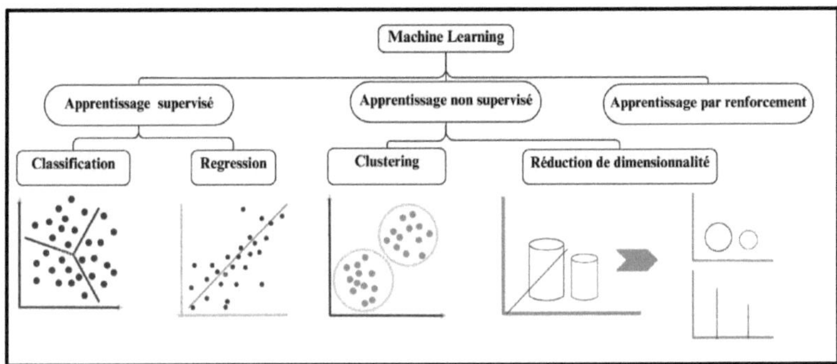


**Figure 7General diagram of *"Machine Learning"* techniques [2]**

### 1.3.1. Supervised learning

In ML, supervised learning involves an automated process carried out through a learning algorithm. This algorithm uses a training dataset, whose target values (the values to be predicted) are known in advance. During the training phase, the perceptron generates an output and compares it to a derived output value provided by the training data. In this way, the model's predictions are compared with these target values in order to fine-tune its parameters. This comparison is carried out using a function that evaluates the magnitude of the model's error. In the event of misclassification, the perceptron then adjusts the weights accordingly **[24]**.

A perceptron, or *"single layer"* perceptron, can be trained solely to perform regression or classification tasks. For each of these tasks, a specific training phase is required. During this training phase, a model is fitted using a set of data for which both inputs and expected responses are known. This means that the model is exposed to a large number of examples where it can learn to make accurate predictions **[18,24].**

The model analyzes the training data and uses a learning algorithm to adjust its internal parameters to minimize the error between the predictions it generates and the actual responses provided in the training data.

#### 1.3.1.1. Classification

The aim of classification is to assign labels or categories to input data according to certain predefined criteria. This data can be of various types, such as patient information or images. This process is often referred to as *"pattern* recognition", and is generally performed through a supervised learning process. **[25].**

In the medical context, this could mean, for example, classifying patients according to their symptoms, or diagnosing a disease based on test results. In the image domain, it could mean identifying specific objects or features in an image **[25].**

Supervised learning involves the use of training data in which the classification labels are already known. The model then learns to associate the characteristics of the data with the corresponding labels, enabling it to classify new data.

Classification aims to automatically determine whether an input is positive or negative according to a predefined criterion. To evaluate the performance of an Artificial Neural Network (ANN) in this task, the so-called "confusion matrix" is often used. **[26]**presented in **Table II**.

**Table IIExample of a confusion matrix for a predictive diagnostic model [26]**

| | | **REALITY**<br>**Whether the patient is affected or not** | |
|---|---|---|---|
| | | Is reached | Not reached |
| **PREDICTION**<br>**What the model predicts** | Is reached | Number of True Positives | Number of False Positives |
| | Not reached | Number of False Negatives | Number of True Negatives |

This matrix quantifies four important criteria, defined as follows:

- True Positive (VP): A positive sample that has been correctly classified as positive.
- False Positive (FP): This is a negative sample that has been incorrectly classified as positive.
- True Negative (TN): A negative sample that has been correctly classified as negative.
- False Negative (FN): A positive sample that has been incorrectly classified as negative.

These four criteria allow us to assess the performance of a classification model by identifying cases where it has correctly or incorrectly classified input data as positive or negative. This gives a precise indication of the model's accuracy and reliability in its classification task **[27]**. The measures used to evaluate the performance of a model are very similar to those used to evaluate the performance of a diagnostic test in medicine. **Table III** details each measure and the corresponding calculation formula.

**Table IIIPerformance indicators for a predictive model: Definition and calculation formulae [28,29]**

| Notion | Definition | Calculation formula |
|---|---|---|
| **Precision** | Proportion of instances predicted as positive that are actually positive | $Précision = \frac{VP}{VP + FP}$ |
| **Sensitivity** | Proportion of real positive instances correctly predicted | $Sensibilité = \frac{VP}{VP + FN}$ |
| **F1score** | Value combining both precision and sensitivity. It is particularly useful when the balance between these two measures is important. | $F1\text{score} = \frac{2 \times Précision \times Sensibilité}{Précision + Sensibilité}$ |
| **Specific** | Proportion of real negative instances correctly predicted | $Spécificité = \frac{VN}{VN + FP}$ |
| **Accuracy** | Proportion of correctly predicted instances among all instances | $Exactitude = \frac{VP + VN}{VP + VN + FP + FN}$ |

#### 1.3.1.2. Regression

Regression in ML is a statistical technique that aims to model and predict a numerical variable as a function of other variables (called explanatory variables or predictors). Unlike classification, where the aim is to categorize data, regression seeks to estimate a continuous quantity **[30]**.

A concrete example of regression would be to predict the disease score as a function of different characteristics such as biological values, age, ... The regression model learns to establish a mathematical relationship between these characteristics and the disease score, enabling accurate predictions to be made for new **cases [27]**.

Regression algorithms are widely used in fields such as economics, finance, medicine, and other sciences where it is essential to make quantitative predictions based on data. Regression methods can vary in complexity, from simple models such as linear regression, which assumes a linear relationship between variables, to more sophisticated models such as neural networks or *random forests*, which can capture complex, non-linear relationships between input data and the variable to be predicted. The choice of method depends on the nature of the data and the complexity of the problem **[31]**.

In linear regression, the relationship between a dependent variable *Y* and one or more independent variables *X* is modeled as a straight line. The general form of the simple linear regression equation **is [31]**:

$$Y = \beta 0 + \beta 1X + \varepsilon$$

- *Y* is the dependent variable,
- *X* is the independent variable,
- $\beta 0$ is the intercept,
- $\beta 1$ is the slope of the line (coefficient),
- $\varepsilon$ is the error term.

The method of least squares is often used to estimate the coefficients $\beta 0$ and $\beta 1$. The formulas for these coefficients in the case of simple linear regression are as follows. **[31]**:

$$\beta 1 = \frac{\sum_{i=1}^{n}(Xi - \bar{X})(Yi - \bar{Y})}{\sum_{i=1}^{n}(Xi - \bar{X})^2}$$

$$\beta 0 = \bar{Y} - \beta 1\bar{X}$$

Where:

- *n* is the number of observations,
- *Xi* and *Yi* are the individual values of *X* and *Y*,
- $\bar{X}$ and $\bar{Y}$ are the means of *X* and *Y* respectively.

Once the coefficients have been estimated, the regression equation can be used to predict the dependent variable $Y$ for new values of $X$ using the regression line, modeled in **Fig. 8 [32]**.

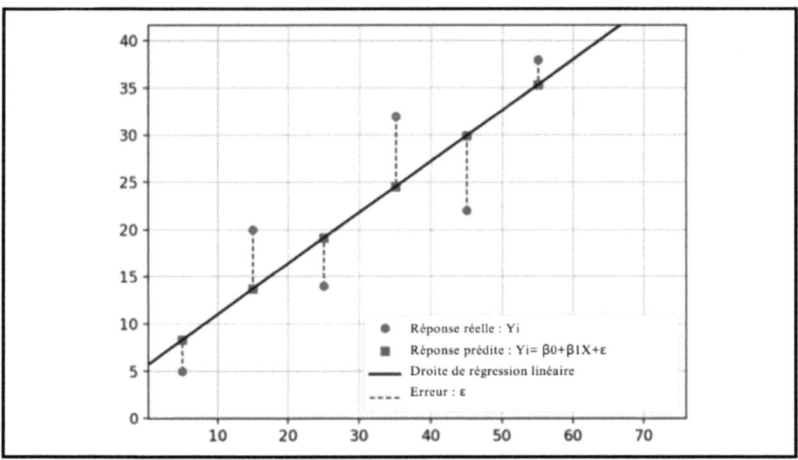


**Figure 8Modeling a simple linear regression [33]**

In the case of multiple regression, where there are several independent variables, the equation becomes **[31]** :

$$Y = \beta 0 + \beta 1X1 + \beta 2X2 + \cdots + \beta kXk + \varepsilon$$

Formulas for coefficients 0, 1, ..., $\beta 0$, $\beta 1$,...,$\beta k$ in the case of multiple regression can be obtained using similar techniques, often using the least-squares matrix **[30]**.

Evaluating the model's goodness of fit involves the use of measures such as the coefficient of determination $R^2$which quantifies the proportion of the variance of the dependent variable explained by the model.

It is important to note that these formulas are specific to linear regression, and other types of regression (non-linear, logistic, etc.) will have different formulas depending on the nature of the model **[30]**.

Generally speaking, supervised learning algorithms are remarkably accurate, but they also have a number of drawbacks:

- Labeling training data is a costly and time-consuming process.
- Overlearning requires a large database with considerable diversity to improve performance
- The training phase requires a significant amount of computing time, which can be a challenge in terms of execution.

### 1.3.2. Unsupervised learning

Unsupervised learning algorithms have the advantage of training on unlabeled data, unlike their supervised counterparts. It should be noted that the preponderance of data collected in artificial intelligence belongs to this category **[8]**.

In the context of unsupervised learning, these models are developed to intrinsically discover structures, relationships or patterns within the data without depending on the existence of prior labels. This approach offers considerable flexibility, eliminating the need for exhaustive annotations for each training instance. Moreover, in the field of artificial intelligence, most real data are not a priori categorized, which makes the use of unsupervised learning methods particularly relevant **[8]**.

Clustering and dimensionality reduction represent two fundamental paradigms in unsupervised learning, each making a distinctive contribution to the analysis of complex data.

#### 1.3.2.1. *"Clustering*

As a method, *clustering* aims to partition a data set into homogeneous groups, known as clusters, as shown in **figure 9**. The underlying idea is to organize the data in such a way that elements within a single cluster are more similar to each other than to elements in other clusters. **[8]**.

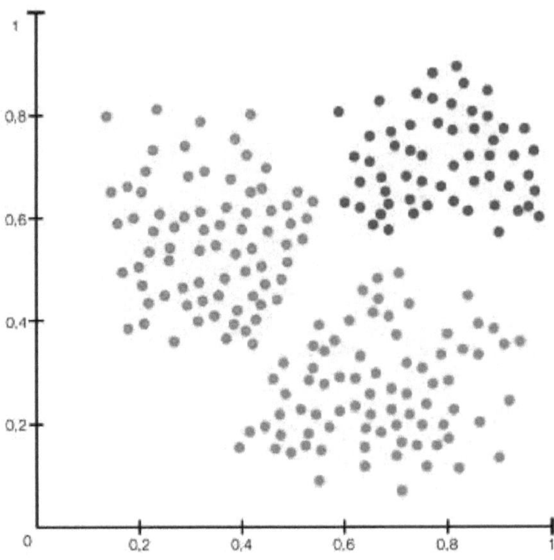


**Figure 9 Example of *clustering* results [34]**

*Clustering* is central to many data-driven bioinformatics investigations and is a powerful computational method. In particular, it helps to analyze unstructured, high-dimensional data in the form of sequences, expressions, texts and images. This is employed with the aim of acquiring data on biological processes at the genomic scale **[35]**.

For example, the clustering of gene expressions offers revealing clues to the natural structure inherent in the data, promoting understanding of gene functions, cellular processes, cell subtypes, and enabling a better apprehension of gene regulations **[35]**.

The fundamental *clustering* algorithm, *"K-means"*, assigns each component of a data set to a single cluster at a time. Data are assigned to the cluster whose centroid is closest; each point is assigned in binary form to a specific cluster **[35]**.

In contrast, the fuzzy *clustering* approach *("Fuzzy c-means"* or FCM ) allows a pixel to belong to several groups with a fuzzy community function value in the range 0 to 1. It is used to partition grayscale and color images, with the flexibility of defining the number of clusters in advance. This method adjusts its objective as needed, making FCM adaptable to different types of images **[36]**.

An improvement of FCM, called *"Kernelized fuzzy C-means"* (KFCM), replaces the Euclidean distance with a kernel-induced separation, offering better noise resistance in the compensation of intensity heterogeneities in magnetic resonance imaging (MRI) images **[36]**.

*Clustering* algorithms, while effective for medium-sized, low-dimensional datasets, encounter accuracy and efficiency difficulties with high-dimensional datasets. High computational complexity can be mitigated by using representation learning in tandem with *clustering*. The use of nonlinear and spectral dimensionality reduction methods is also advocated to achieve improved *"clustering"* results without losing essential information **[36]**.

#### 1.3.2.2. Dimensionality reduction

The aim of dimensionality reduction is to reduce the number of features or variables in a dataset, while preserving as much of the crucial information as possible. This approach becomes essential when the original data are characterized by intrinsic complexity and a large number of dimensions **[25]**. Various dimensionality reduction techniques can be used:

- Principal Component Analysis (PCA) : This seeks to identify the main axes, shown in **Figure 10**, along which the data vary the most. By projecting the data onto these axes, we can represent the whole dataset with a reduced number of dimensions, while preserving a large part of the variance. **[37]**.

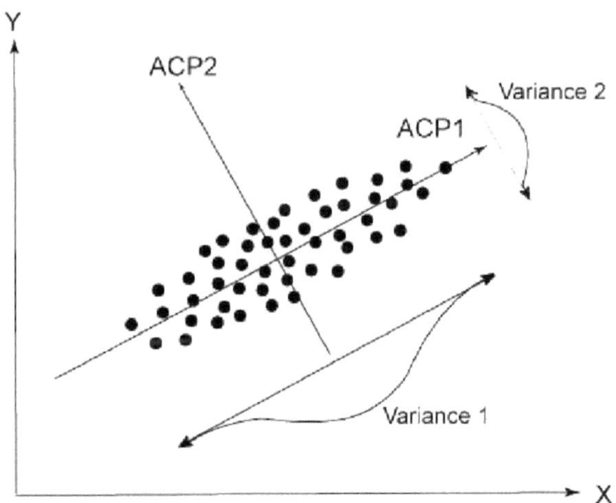


**Figure 10 Variance reduction along the principal axes [38]**

- *"t-Distributed Stochastic Neighbor Embedding (*T-SNE): This is a dimensionality reduction method used primarily for visualization. It seeks to preserve similarity relationships between points, thus facilitating the graphical representation of data in a reduced-dimension space. **[37]**.
- Auto-encoders: these are neural networks that learn to represent data in a compressed way. They consist of an encoding phase where information is reduced, followed by a decoding phase to reconstruct the original data. This facilitates analysis, visualization and helps alleviate the problems associated with the "curse of dimensionality." **[8]**.

### 1.3.3. Reinforcement learning

Reinforcement learning ( *"Reinforcement Learning"*, RL ) is a branch of ML concerned with learning sequential actions in an environment in order to maximize a notion of cumulative reward **[2]**. Unlike supervised learning, where the model is trained on labeled data, and unsupervised learning, which explores the intrinsic structures of the data, reinforcement learning relies on the idea of dynamic interaction with an environment to learn how to make optimal decisions **[8]**.

This type of learning is based on key elements (**Figure 11**) **[39]**:

- Agent: The entity that makes decisions in an environment. It can be an algorithm, an AI, or even a human being in certain applications.
- Environment : The context in which the agent evolves. This can be virtual (as in video games) or real (as in robotics).
- State: The current state of the environment, which influences the agent's possible actions.
- Action: The decision taken by the agent at a given moment. Actions can have consequences for the environment.
- Reward: A numerical signal that evaluates the quality of the action taken by the agent. The agent's objective is to maximize the cumulative reward over time.
- Policy: The strategy or plan the agent follows to choose its actions based on the current state of the environment.

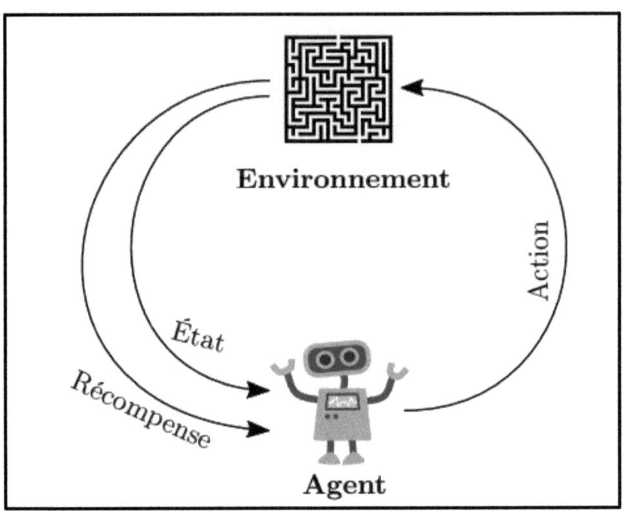


**Figure 11Illustration of the general framework of reinforcement learning [39]**

The reinforcement learning process takes place through cycles of interaction between the agent and the environment, as shown in **figure 12**. The agent takes an action according to its policy, observes the resulting state and the associated reward, then adjusts its policy to maximize future rewards. This iterative process allows the agent to learn to make more efficient decisions over time, by exploring different actions and adjusting its policy according to the results obtained **[40]**.

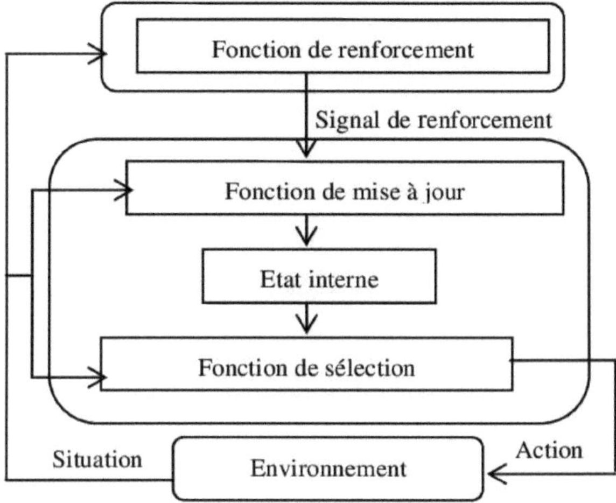


**Figure 12 :Reinforcement learning process [41]**

Reinforcement learning has demonstrated its effectiveness in large-scale text generation, notably with models such as *"Generative pre-trained transformer"* (GPT) **[42]**. However, its application can be tedious due to computational complexity and stability issues. In contexts where strict constraints are required, the RL approach may not be the most suitable. **[40]**.

### 1.4.Main areas of artificial intelligence

The specific characteristics of a domain are closely linked to the format of its input and output data. Each domain has its own requirements in terms of the types of data it handles. For example, in data science, structured data, whether numerical or categorical, comes from a variety of sources such as Excel files or databases, feeding into statistical analysis, predictive modeling and data-driven decision-making. In *natural* language *processing* (NLP), textual data predominates, directing tasks towards language understanding, machine translation and sentiment analysis. Conversely, in computer vision, visual data, in the form of images, are essential for tasks such as facial recognition, image segmentation and object detection **[8]**.

### 1.4.1. Data Science

Data Science focuses on the acquisition, storage, processing and analysis of large quantities of data. In the context of AI, Data Science plays a crucial role in preparing data for ML models. This includes data mining, pattern detection and the creation of predictive models. AI models can be used to predict future events based on historical trends. This is particularly useful in demand forecasting, resource planning and strategic decision-making. Regression, classification and *"clustering"*, are often used in Data Science to derive useful knowledge from data **[43]**.

### 1.4.2. Automatic natural language processing

NLP concerns the ability of machines to understand, interpret and generate human language in a natural way. NLP applications include language understanding, machine translation, text generation, automatic summarization and sentiment analysis. Recent advances in NLP, particularly with the use of pre-trained language models such as *"Transformers"*, have greatly improved the ability of machines to understand and generate complex natural language. AI can be used to understand and process human language, enabling the analysis of large amounts of textual data, such as customer reviews, medical documents, or posts on social networks **[42]**.

### 1.4.3. Computer vision

Computer Vision aims to enable machines to understand and interpret visual information from images or videos. This includes object detection, facial recognition, image segmentation, image classification, and many other applications **[25]**.

Machine learning techniques, in particular DL, have considerably improved the performance of computer vision systems. These models can learn to automatically represent relevant features from visual data. Computer vision algorithms use techniques such as CNNs to extract meaningful features from images, enabling machines to make decisions based on visual information **[25]**.

These fields often interact with each other, forming complete AI systems. For example, in Data Science, machine learning models can be applied to textual datasets (NLP) or visual data (Computer Vision) to extract richer, more complex information. Integrating these fields helps create more sophisticated and versatile AI systems **[8]**.

# 2. ADVANCES IN ARTIFICIAL INTELLIGENCE FOR HEMATOLOGY

AI is essentially based on the acquisition and use of data. In the case of supervised learning, these data are annotated by experts in the field concerned, such as biologists. This helps to guide the model in its learning process by providing it with labeled examples. However, for other applications, such as unsupervised *clustering*, the data may be unlabeled (**Figure 13**). This type of learning generally takes place in two distinct phases: first, data learning, where the model learns to identify structures or patterns in the data without the aid of labels, then comes the inference phase, where the model is ready to be used to perform specific tasks on new data. This approach enables autonomous exploration and discovery of the information contained in unlabeled data, thus offering great flexibility in the analysis and interpretation of results **[44]**.

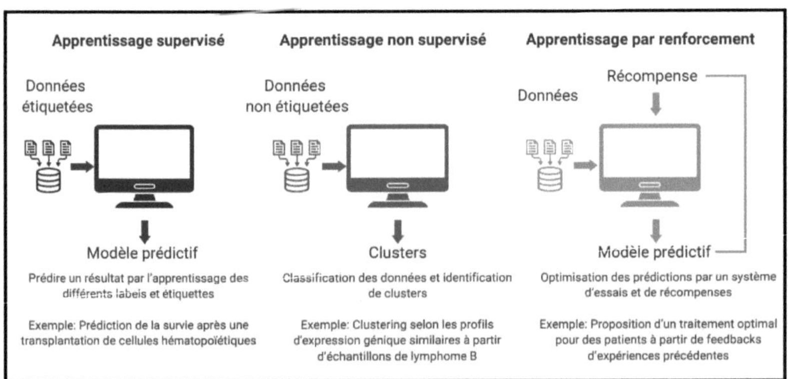


**Figure 13 The three types of *Machine Learning* models and examples of prediction in the medical field [44]**

Before embarking on a review of innovative applications in laboratory hematology, it's worth pointing out that the automation currently taken for granted is based on the prior use of AI systems integrated into clinical practice. These systems first became integrated by being implemented in medical analysis laboratories to perform biological diagnosis and facilitate its interpretation. The first applications of AI in this field involved the detection of cells by image analysis and automatic cell counting by hematology automatons. Subsequently, AI came to play an important role in hematology prediction and therapeutic guidance in clinical hematology.

### 2.1.Medical image analysis: AI-assisted diagnosis

Blood cell analysis is the starting point for the diagnosis of 80% of haematological diseases. **[45]**. Quantitative morphological analysis can therefore assist cytologists in the evaluation of blood and bone marrow samples and enable conclusions to be drawn about the patient's condition. Nevertheless, these procedures are complex and time-consuming, involving a specialist scrutinizing the sample through a microscope, thus exposing the process to potential human error. In recent years, various initiatives have been undertaken to automate these procedures using image processing and machine learning techniques, making the process faster and more cost-effective, while significantly reducing the workload in laboratories **[17]**. CNNs, known to provide excellent results in image recognition tasks, have been the subject of much research with a view to their application in hematology cytology.

The integration of artificial intelligence in the analysis of medical images for diagnosis includes, first and foremost, the detection, quantification and morphological evaluation of cells. In particular, it includes the use of flow cytometry and multi-omics data analysis in the precise identification and classification of cell populations and their immunophenotypic profiles, facilitating reliable recognition of biological profiles **[44]**.

### 2.1.1. Detection, counting and evaluation of cell morphology

Using imaging and image processing techniques, AI can isolate cells in a sample, identify them based on their morphology, and provide precision counting. Models can be trained on large datasets to recognize different cell types, adapting to the morphological variability present in biological samples **[46]**.

#### 2.1.1.1. Steps

AI recognition of blood cells involves several complex steps to classify, count and study the morphology of the blood's figurative elements.

❖ **Image segmentation and pre-processing**

The first step is to segment the image to isolate the blood cells from the rest of the image by dividing it into different non-overlapping parts. These parts are called *"Region of interest"* (ROI). While the human visual system naturally segments images without any particular effort, automatic segmentation is one of the most complex tasks in image processing and computer vision **[47]**.

In the case of peripheral blood cells, segmentation aims to separate the whole cell from the background, and also to separate its main components. Most works consider two ROIs: the nucleus and the cytoplasm **[48]**. If we consider a digital color image as a grid of rectangular pixels, the color images are decomposed into several grayscale images according to a color model. Pixels are then described quantitatively by a number representing light intensity on a continuous scale between 0 (black) and a maximum (white) **[47]**.

The end result of any segmentation method is a set of binary images, commonly referred to as masks. Each mask contains a single ROI visualized by a limited white region on a black background (**Figure 14**) **[48]**.

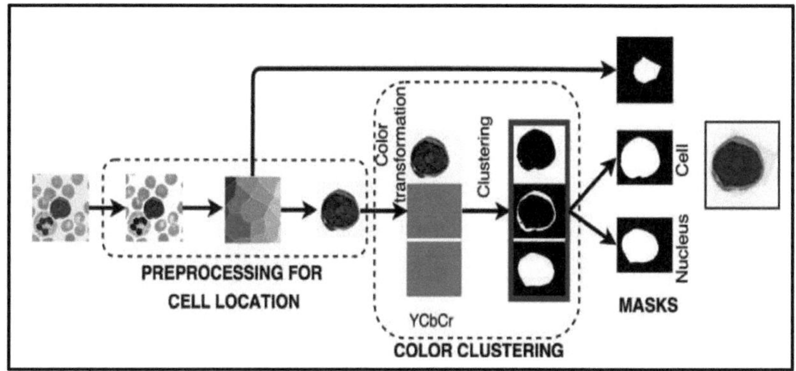


**Figure 14Two-step image segmentation process to obtain three *"Regions Of Interest"* from a blood cell image. [48]**

Segmentation algorithms have been applied in previous work to distinguish normal leukocytes from blast cells in blood and bone marrow. However, segmentation of atypical lymphocytes is limited and complex due to morphological variability. Unlike normal cells, where segmentation is facilitated by distinct features, atypical cells require a more elaborate approach to extract specific characteristics **[48]**. This underlines the need to develop advanced methods to improve their detection and characterization in hematology, while taking into account other clinical and biological parameters.

❖ **Feature extraction**

After the segmentation stage, feature extraction takes place. This involves the identification of quantitative descriptors in each ROI mask, grouped into three main categories: geometric, colored and textured. These three feature categories are described in **Table** IV **[48]**.

**Table IVDescription of the three categories of features to be extracted from masks [45,48]**

| Category | Features | Description |
|---|---|---|
| **Geometry** | Perimeter, shape of nucleus and cytoplasm | Measurement of cell shape, size and regularity: important parameters for visual observation by pathologists. |
| **Color** | Color histograms, first-order statistics | Analysis of the distribution of color intensity values in the image, to extract statistical parameters such as mean, standard deviation and entropy. |
| **Texture** | Particle size distribution, particle size curves | Evaluation of particle size distribution and cell texture, providing information on internal cell composition and structure. |

This additional information provides a quantitative representation of the visual appearance of cells, integrating morphological and colorimetric aspects for a complete analysis.

❖ **Numerical classification**

After segmentation and feature extraction, each cell image is uniquely represented by a set of numerical descriptors. Automatic classification aims to assign this set of descriptors to a specific cell class from a set of known classes. The classifier, as a system designed for this task, is based on a mathematical model whose structure and parameters must be adjusted correctly **[47]**.

Model training is supervised, using a training set of images identified by pathologists. Model validation is performed on a separate set of images not used in training, which can be achieved by separating the image sets or by a cross-validation approach. Commonly employed methods for blood cell classification include neural networks and decision trees **[44]**.

#### 2.1.1.2. Applications

AI can therefore be trained to recognize different blood cell types using large datasets. This ability enables it to distinguish and count cells accurately, speeding up the cell counting process and reducing reliance on manual methods.

- **Automatic reading of blood smear slides**

  - Haematological laboratory work-up

The combination of microscopic image digitization and AI enables automated image processing and cell differentiation, reducing the need for human intervention. Traditional methods involved complex pre-processing steps to distinguish artifacts from informative elements prior to cell classification. In contrast, with recent ML-based systems, the steps are less strictly separated, trusting the algorithm to automatically detect cells and extract relevant and significant features for accurate cell labeling. Although automated hematology analyzers remain indispensable in hematology laboratories, interferences and pathological conditions still require manual verification. Fortunately, digitization of peripheral blood smears and quantification of blood cell lineages based on machine-learning models sometimes enable computers to provide their opinion on these smear slides before anyone has examined a cell **[1,48]**.

One of the best examples of an automated microscope for reading blood smear slides is the CellaVision® range of systems, which uses an ML model to classify blood smear observations into one of 17 cell types, including mature and immature forms (**Figure 15**) **[46]**.

Based on a smear stained with de May-Grünwald Giemsa (MGG) stain, the software performs morphological recognition and classification into 12 leukocyte populations: mature neutrophils, eosinophils, basophils, lymphocytes, monocytes, promyelocytes, myelocytes, metamyelocytes, plasma cells, blast cells tricholeukocytes and atypical lymphocytes. Unidentified cells, erythroblasts, giant thrombocytes, thrombocyte agglutinations, Sézary cells and artefacts are added to these categories. The saving in analysis time is estimated at around 30% compared with manual recognition and counting, but the system is not designed to verify results independently of a trained operator **[46]**.

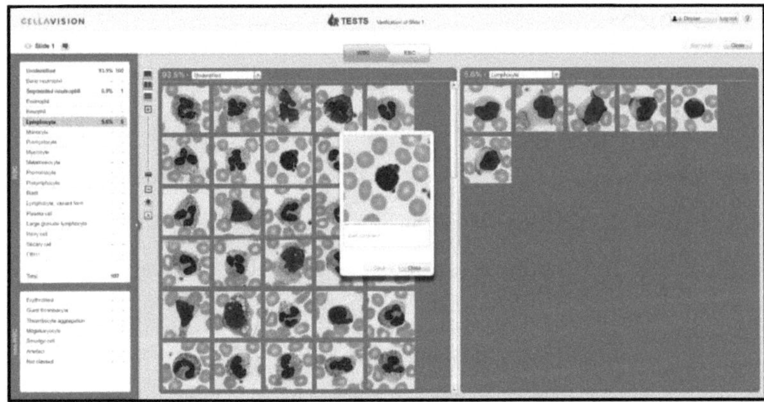


**Figure 15Example of blood smear cell classification using CellaVision® prior to expert validation. [49]**

Although leukocyte counting is mastered by CellaVision® with a specificity of over 96%, red cell counting remains limited by the need for a greater number of large fields. This explains the specificity of 58.3% for the analysis of red blood cells, and in particular acanthocytes and schizocytes **[50]**thus limiting its use for the diagnosis of microangiopathic hemolytic anemia in hemolytic uremic syndrome according to *"International Committee for Standardization of Hematology"* (ICSH) **[46,50]**.

Further work led to the Scopio Labs X100® system, which overcame the limits of red cell and platelet detection and counting. Full-field red cell evaluation was measured with an accuracy of 96.29% and a specificity of 97.62%, while platelet estimation was evaluated at 94.89% for accuracy and 96.28% for specificity. The system enabled full-field analysis of peripheral blood smears from previously prepared slides **[51]**visible in **figure 16**.

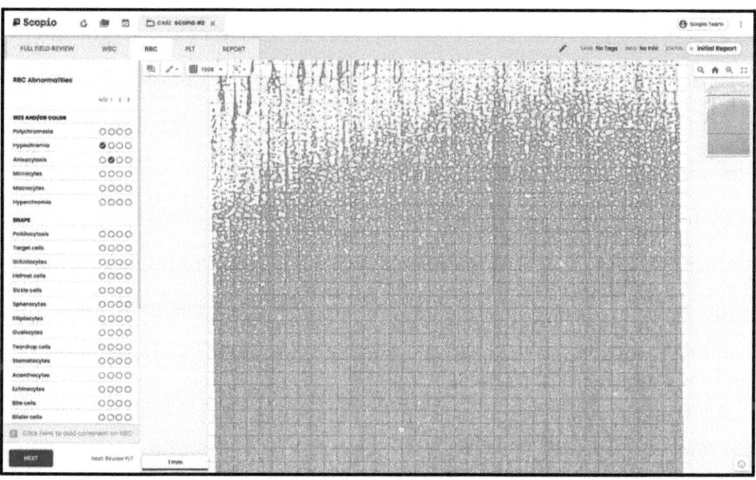


**Figure 16Detailed analysis of red cell abnormalities in full field on the Scopio Labs X100® automated system [52]**

Another AI-assisted blood cell analysis system, the Mantiscope®, uses AI to fully classify blood cells and detect abnormalities. This in vitro diagnostics system consists of a scanner coupled to a *"cloud"*, which is a collaborative data storage space. The blood smear is automatically digitized by the scanner. The system then analyzes the smear samples after uploading the images to the cloud based on the patient's barcode. Healthcare professionals can modify the template's recommendations using the system's annotation interface **[52]**.

To further reduce the time required for analysis, and the dependence on human resources within the laboratory, robotics and ML techniques have even made it possible to spread and color slides for analysis. Roche's COBAS M511® illustrates the possibilities of fully image-based hematology analysis, exploring the full range of blood count parameters from cells "printed" and stained on a slide. The instrument can provide both quantitative and morphological information simultaneously, eliminating the need for slide preparation, stains and reagents, thus reducing space requirements. A multicenter validation study demonstrated good correlation of standard parameters and alerts with reference methods of 96%, although precise data on the accuracy of individual cell classification were not provided **[53]**.

Researchers are now focusing on the detection of increasingly complex immature forms, morphological variants and pathological morphotypes. Various machine-learning approaches have produced encouraging results in the identification and differentiation of myeloid blasts, lymphoblasts and promyelocytes individually, as well as all three simultaneously. Pathological forms such as atypical lymphocytes and mature lymphoid neoplasms have also been studied.

The Mindray MC-80® locates and pre-classifies cells in blood smears, and boasts 93.6% sensitivity for reactive lymphocytes, with a negative predictive value equal to 97.8%. This model also detects immature granulocytes, neoplastic cells and nucleated red blood cells **[54]**.

**Figure 17** shows images of blasts observed in the blood smear of a patient with acute myeloid leukemia, showing Auer bodies (A), immature granulation (B) and cup-like nucleoli (C). Dysplastic eosinophils are also seen in a patient with myelodysplastic syndrome (D), and atypical lymphocytes observed in three patients with lymphoid neoplasms (E, follicular lymphoma; F, Hairy Cell Leukemia; G, Sézary syndrome). The model also detects plasma cells observed in a patient with plasma cell leukemia (H) and cells observed in the peripheral blood of patients with infections (I, neutrophil with Plasmodium-derived Maurer spot in cytoplasm; J, malaria parasites inside an erythrocyte; K, leishmaniasis parasites in the cytoplasm of a neutrophil) **[55]**.

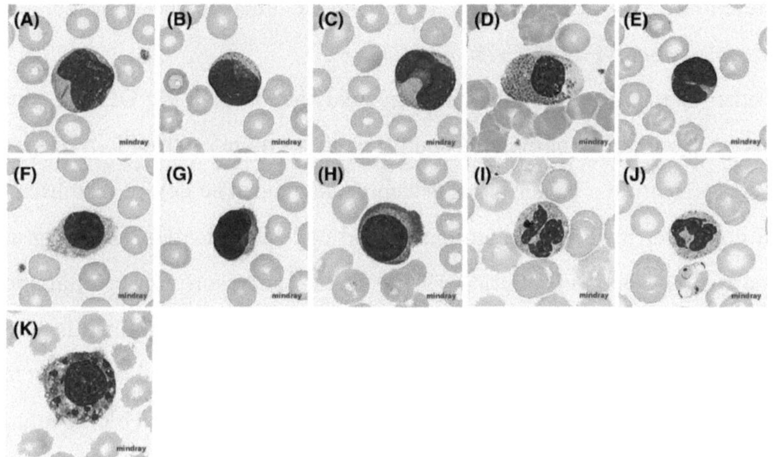


**Figure 17Images of atypical cells provided by Mindray MC-80® [55]**

Although hematological cell analysis is an important first step in the diagnosis of hematological malignancies, a complete and accurate diagnosis often requires a combination of different complementary techniques and analyses.

- Bedside hematology workup

What's more, in addition to laboratory analyzers, machine learning-based hematology has also made inroads into community care, also known as *"Point Of Care"* (PoC).

A portable point-of-care complete cell blood count analyzer, the PixCell HemoScreen®, has been compared to traditional hematology analyzers.

Using computer vision AI technology, it bridges the gap in bedside diagnostics. Researchers concluded that it can deliver laboratory-equivalent results quickly and accurately, making it an alternative for improving workflows and minimizing the spread of disease. Compared with traditional analysis methods, it differs from conventional methods in its ability to better differentiate between cells and better handle interference from standard hematology analyzers **[56,57]**.

Another example of PoC's hematology analyzers is Le Sight OLO®, which delivers laboratory-quality cell count results in minutes from two drops of blood taken from a finger prick or venous sample. The device also uses AI and computer imaging to automate blood cell identification, counting and abnormality detection, offering 19 parameters and more powerful atypical cell reporting capabilities. The Sight OLO® has received approval from the *"Food and Drug Administration"* (FDA) for a complete blood cell count test with a finger prick sample, requiring only 5% of the minimum blood volume needed for traditional laboratory equipment while providing the same quality of results **[56]**.

The analyzer shown in **figure 18** measures approximately 30x25x30cm (A) and consists of a single-use test kit (B) (1, cartridge; 2, mixing tube; 3, dropper cap; 4, microcapillary). The sample is taken at the fingertip (C) and analysis shows falsely colored micrographs collected using OLO multispectral microscopy for different types of white blood cells (D) or others (E). The red channel reflects hemoglobin uptake, the green channel illustrates deoxyribonucleic acid (DNA) fluorescence and the blue channel is cytoplasmic staining.

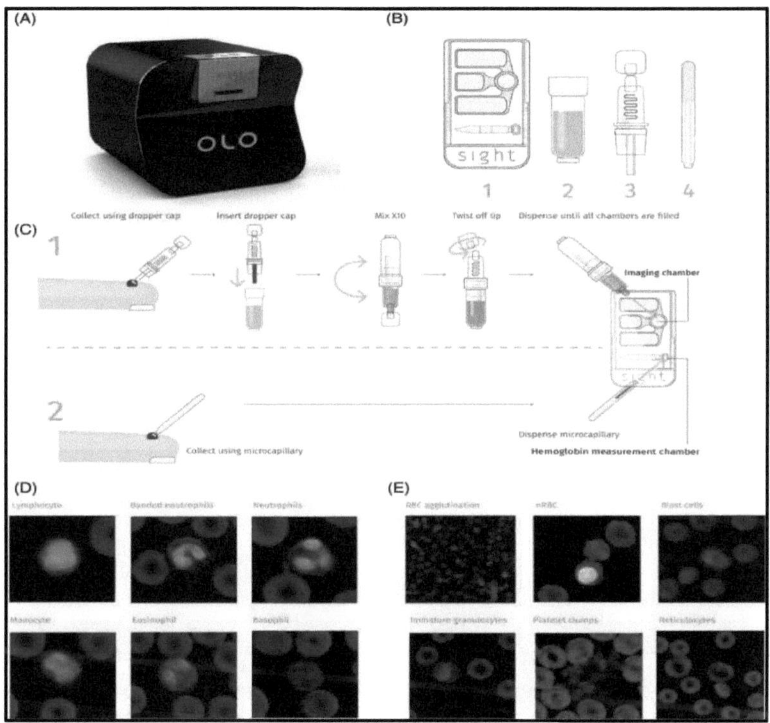


**Figure 18The Sight OLO® haematological analysis system [56]**

Currently, patients at risk of febrile neutropenia due to cancer chemotherapy, idiosyncratic drug reactions or congenital disorders are monitored in hospital or clinical laboratories. For many patients, effective and frequent monitoring is difficult because of the time required and the cost of repeated laboratory visits. Athelas One®, a miniature hematology analyzer, has been developed for home monitoring of white blood cells and neutrophils in particular. A drop of blood (~ 3.5 μL) taken from the finger or from an anticoagulated blood sample is placed on a specially designed strip, to create a precisely sized layer of blood cells. The slide is then inserted into the device, which analyzes the test strip on the basis of an image analysis process **[58]**. By comparing the results with a standard laboratory counter, the Sysmex XE5000®, the FDA approves the equivalence of the two methods through linear regression (**Figure 19**) **[59]**.

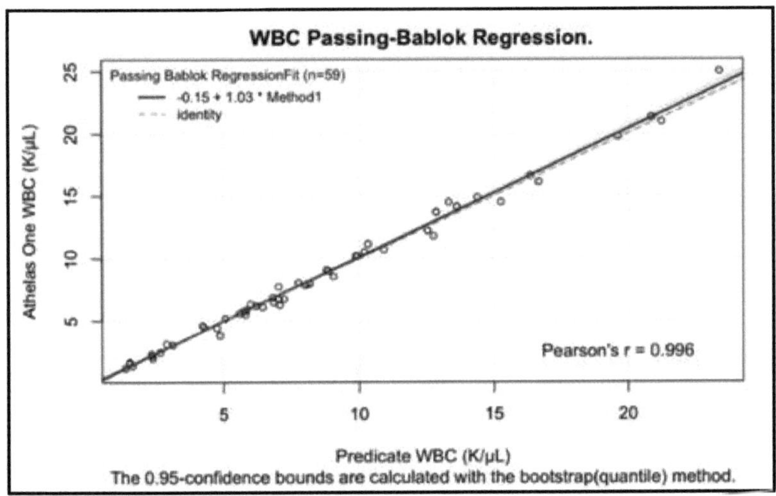


**Figure 19Linear regression explaining the concordance of leukocyte count results between Athelas One® and Sysmex XE5000®. [59]**

- **Bone marrow smear**

The myelogram, used to evaluate the cellular composition of the bone marrow (BM), is indispensable for detecting hematological abnormalities, particularly in leukemia and disorders of central origin. Morphogo® is an AI-assisted BM smear analysis system that can differentiate nucleated cells into specific categories and provide useful diagnostic information. It uses a 27-layer CNN that captures multiple high-resolution images of the medullary smear and stitches them together to generate a complete image of the target morphology. The CNN's convolution layer can improve the image quality of the cell group by eliminating or highlighting specific cell features during image processing, such as blurring and edging. Blood cell group characteristics are extracted and classified as leukemic or non-leukemic. Morphogo®'s performance in identifying hematological lineage cells in 230 cases gave a classification accuracy of 85.7 to 91%. The average sensitivity and specificity of the system were 69.4% and 97.2% respectively **[46]**. Classification of 68610 bone marrow nucleated cell images by the Morphogo® system compared with that of pathologists demonstrated almost perfect concordance **(Figure 20) [60]**.

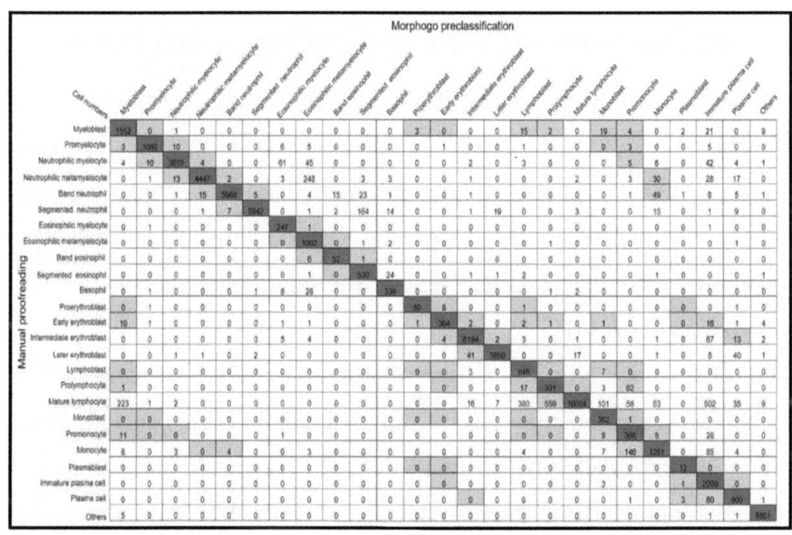


**Figure 20:Classification of cellular images using Morphogo® system pre-ranking and manual verification [60]**

The confusion matrix in **Fig. 20** shows the number of cell images assigned to each of the 25 morphological categories of bone marrow nucleated cells. The rows indicate the results of the Morphogo® system pre-classification, while the columns represent the results of verification by pathologists. The diagonal boxes in the matrix indicate the number of cell classifications consistent with both the Morphogo® system and the pathologists. Confusions considered tolerable are highlighted in light blue.

Another study showed that Morphogo® had 82% accuracy and 91% specificity in identifying metastatic cancer cells compared to pathologists. Therefore, it is thought that Morphogo® has potential as an AI tool for MO smear analysis in the future, possibly obviating the need for additional analyses such as flow cytometry and molecular analysis **[46]**.

### 2.1.2. Flow cytometry and immunophenotypic data analysis

Multiparametric flow cytometry (FMC) and immunohistology are essential elements in the routine diagnosis and monitoring of hematological diseases through the analysis of cell populations. FMC uses monoclonal antibodies conjugated to fluorescent dyes, targeting specific antigens, to analyze cell populations according to their light-scattering properties and antigenic expression patterns **[61]**.

Modern flow cytometers can analyze thousands of cells per second, and can also assess hematopoietic cells at the individual level, generating large multidimensional data sets that are difficult for humans to interpret directly. The technology converts fluorescence signals into electrical pulses, which are then digitized and stored in a standardized file format. The files contain a matrix of expression values for all fluorescent dyes measured for all particles analyzed by a flow cytometer. Accompanying software pre-processes and visualizes the data to facilitate analysis by human experts. Expression values are typically displayed as two-dimensional graphs, and a sequential sorting procedure is applied to identify and label cell populations of interest **[62]**.

Quality management systems are in place to standardize laboratory processes such as sample preparation and measurement, but data analysis and interpretation remain the responsibility of humans, relying entirely on expert knowledge with inherent inter-observer variability **[63]**. In order to reduce reliance on expert knowledge and potentially increase the consistency of data interpretation, the implementation of automated processes is necessary. Researchers have recently reviewed typical developments and applications of machine learning in CMF, providing an overview of the basic knowledge of intelligent imaging CMF **[62]**.

In automated analysis of CMF data, most machine-learning-based models include an additional pre-processing step converting expression values into images prior to the segmentation step discussed above.

Examples include the use of algorithms to differentiate acute myeloid leukemia from healthy samples based on graphs of CMF data in two dimensions (2D ) which were transformed into image files. A weighted value was assigned to each pixel in the images, then reduced to a binary array. The use of self-organizing maps as input to a CNN enabled the distinction between healthy and neoplastic samples, as well as the classification of subtypes of mature B neoplasms. One study involving blood or bone marrow samples showed that a CNN classified all eight B lymphoma subtypes with a confidence of at least 0.95, achieving a weighted F1 score of 0.94 **[61]**. Features learned from the original model were used to train models for different CMF protocols, facilitating their deployment in routine diagnostic environments.

In the case of minimal residual disease detection in acute myeloid leukemia, CMF data can be analyzed by machine learning algorithms to identify cancer cells remaining after treatment. Studies have shown that these algorithms can achieve diagnostic accuracy comparable to that of human experts **[64]**.

Like machine-learning-based image analysis, automated cytometry has the potential to automate and standardize existing techniques, thereby increasing efficiency and reducing human error. However, to determine which approach is most appropriate in the context of CMF laboratories, several factors must be taken into account, such as patient and disease characteristics, performance, as well as IT infrastructure and costs **[65]**.

### 2.1.3. Multi-omics analysis

With the growing importance of genetic factors in the diagnosis, prognosis and treatment selection of hematological malignancies, considerable efforts are being made to redefine subgroups based on pathophysiological mechanisms. Unsupervised learning can be used for exploratory analysis of unlabeled data to infer underlying factors and understand their interactions. Unlike supervised learning, there is no predefined outcome, and results require manual evaluation to estimate the value of identified groups by relating them to clinical and/or genetic factors **[66]**.

Cytogenetics is crucial for identifying chromosomal abnormalities in hematological neoplasms, currently using chromosome band analysis as the reference standard. This provides important information for stratification and prognosis of pathologies, as well as for therapeutic choice. However, the manual karyotyping process is laborious, requiring chromosome detection, segmentation and classification. Automated karyotyping systems are being developed to speed up this process. Chromosome segmentation involves the detection and separation of chromosomes from the metaphase image for accurate classification. DL-based approaches have been used, such as the customized U-Net auto-encoder architecture which has been widely used for segmentation and denoising of **complex** medical images **[67]**. Chromosome classification assigns a position in the karyogram based on features such as shape, size, centromere location and banding pattern. Features are often extracted by CNN, showing promising results. To detect chromosomal abnormalities, numerical classifications are easily extended, but classification of structural abnormalities remains a challenge, although some advances have been made with CNNs such as the chromosome abnormality detection system, called *"Chromosome-Recurrent Abnormality Detector"* (Chromosome-ReAD) . Recent advances suggest that automated karyotyping systems will soon be the norm, facilitating the daily work of cytogeneticists and speeding up the decision-making process **[67]**.

With the democratization of technologies such as next-generation DNA and ribonucleic acid (RNA) sequencing , it is becoming increasingly feasible to obtain personalized data on complex diseases. Machine learning promises to help unravel these data, with many existing bioinformatics tools themselves incorporating machine learning. In proteomics, machine learning models have successfully diagnosed multiple myeloma via mass spectrometry using only peripheral plasma **[68]**. In the context of genomics, RNA sequencing, known as scRNA-seq, has been used to accurately identify gene expression signatures and hematopoietic progenitors visualized in clusters in **figure** 21 **[69]**.

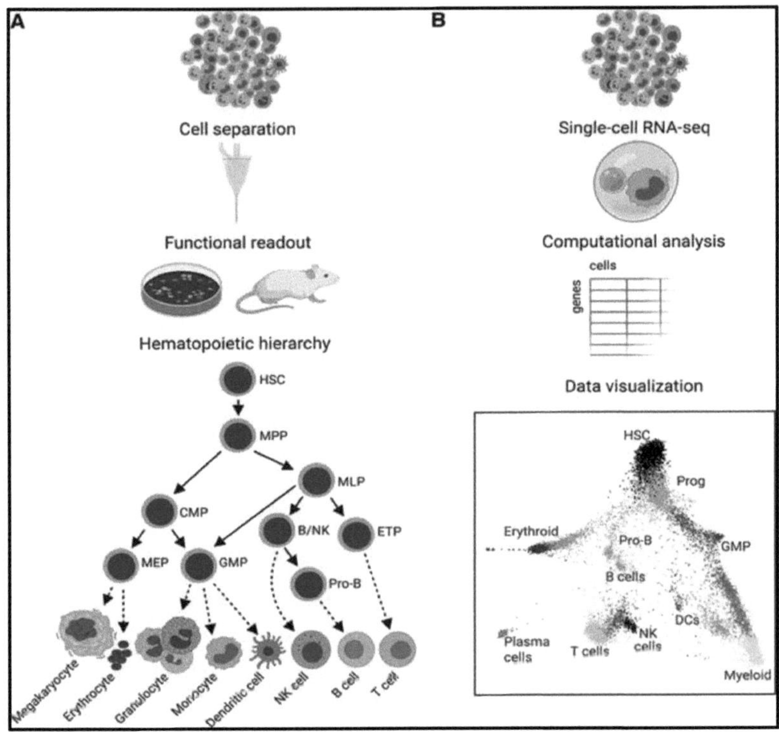


**Figure 21Two approaches to describing the hematopoietic hematopoietic hierarchy [31]**

Hematopoietic cell types can be separated, for example, using flow cytometry based on surface markers (**Figure 21-A).** In vitro differentiation and transplantation in guinea pigs provide information on the lineage of individual cells or sorted populations. These tests have played a major role in establishing hierarchical relationships between cell types.

Molecular characterization of individual cells by RNA sequencing (**Figure 21 - B**) offers an additional method for studying cellular heterogeneity.

Computational analysis of these datasets indicates that cell types are more heterogeneous and differentiation trajectories are more gradual than previously glimpsed **[31]**.

The same technique has been used to predict complete remission after induction therapy for acute myeloid leukemia. Machine learning has also helped predict sensitivities to different therapies in acute myeloid leukemia based on next-generation DNA and RNA sequencing and in vitro drug sensitivity testing **[70]**.

### 2.2. Predicting clinical outcomes and early detection of hematological diseases

Several attempts at an intelligent classification of hematological diseases using blood characteristics are present in the literature. Most of these approaches focus on a binary classification between healthy individuals and patients with a specific disease, or between two specific diseases. These methods have been developed using more traditional machine learning algorithms such as decision trees or *"multilayer"* perceptrons **[71]**. In particular, the last five years have seen the emergence of the use of CNNs to identify hematological malignancies and study the histopathological features of lymphomas (**Table V**).

**Table VStudies of artificial intelligence models used to detect myeloid and lymphoid leukemias**

| **Applications of AI models for the detection of myeloid leukemia** | | | |
|---|---|---|---|
| Study | Input | Output (Pathology) | Performance assessment |
| Matek et al. 2019 **[72]** | Microscopic images of blood smears | LAM | 94% sensitivity |
| Boldu et al. 2019 **[73]** | Colored blood smear | LAM, LAL | Accuracy 85.8% |
| Matek et al. 2021 **[74]** | Images of bone marrow smears | Hematological malignancies | Accuracy > 90%. |
| **Applications of AI models for the detection of lymphoid leukemia** | | | |
| El Achi et al. 2019 **[75]** | Microscopic images of blood smears | Lymphomas | 95% accuracy |
| Sahlol et al. 2020 **[76]** | Hematoxylin and eosin-stained microscope images of lymph node biopsy slides | LAL | Accuracy 97.1% |
| Mohlam et al. 2020 **[77]** | | Large-cell B lymphoma | Accuracy 94 |
| Syrykh et al. 2020 **[78]** | | Follicular lymphoma | AUC 0.99 |

***AML:** Acute myeloid leukemia; **ALL:** Acute lymphocytic leukemia, **AUC:** Area Under Curve (sensitivity vs. 1- specificity curve)*

### 2.2.1. Identifying cancer pathologies

In the case of automatic recognition of acute leukemias, the classification problem is doubly complex. Firstly, it is necessary to differentiate between blast cells and mature cells, as they share certain morphological similarities such as nucleoli, basophilic cytoplasm and fine chromatin. Secondly, it is necessary to distinguish the lymphoid lineage from the myeloid lineage, as they show similar patterns. This problem has rarely been addressed in the literature, although automated blood image analyzers tend to underestimate the number of blasts, confusing them with mature normal cells **[48]**.

AI tools for decision support in oncology are already available. A model has recently been developed to provide a list of probable diagnoses based on age and laboratory measurements, which serve as input to a support vector machine model that is a supervised machine learning technique used for classification and regression **[79]**.

The diagnostic capabilities of machine learning extend to the precise classification of diseases such as acute myeloid leukemia, and to the accurate differentiation between myelodysplastic syndromes and bone marrow aplasia **[14]**. In resource-limited settings, CNN-based diagnostic tools could be invaluable for triage and classification **[80]**.

For diseases with high rates of inter-observer variability (e.g. myelodysplastic syndromes), machine learning-based predictions could provide an additional data point to consider in the event of disagreement or ambiguity. In such cases, the need to establish a reference standard poses a dilemma, as it diminishes the reliability of the labels used to train the machine learning model in the first place.

Results from peripheral blood smears or bone marrow biopsies provide additional information for machine learning-based diagnosis. This information may involve the diagnosis itself, or the distinction between diseases such as chronic lymphocytic leukemia and peripheral lymphoma on the basis of blood counts **[81]**. Work has also shown the usefulness of integrating blood counts with other clinical and genomic data to improve diagnostic accuracy, particularly in the differential diagnosis of bone marrow failure diseases **[82]**.

AI can be used to scrutinize these data and identify complex patterns. For example, algorithms can detect specific genetic mutations associated with certain leukemias, facilitating early diagnosis. An AI-based cytogenetic model identified a correlation between a specific form of myelodysplasia, linked to mutations in the SF3B1 gene encoding the splicing factor, and particular features observed on the peripheral blood smear **[83]**.

### 2.2.2. Histopathology of hematopoietic disorders

DL techniques are increasingly stimulating diagnostic support tools based on image analysis. For example, one algorithm has accurately distinguished between diffuse large B-cell lymphoma and Burkitt's lymphoma, based on raw images of hematoxylin and eosin-stained tissue sections fed into a CNN. Similar algorithms have also been used to identify neoplastic cells in bone marrow aspirates (**Table V**) **[77]**.

In addition, one study used unsupervised learning techniques to detect patterns of organ damage in chronic graft-versus-host disease **[84]**.

## 2.3. Prognostic value and risk stratification of hematological complications

Studies of prognostic markers and treatments for blood cancers have traditionally been conducted on the basis of microscopically defined disease entities, in accordance with the classification guidelines of the World Health Organization (WHO) **[85]**. However, diagnostic ambiguity remains a regular occurrence, and the quality of results largely depends on the experience and skills of the operator. To reduce reliance on expertise and potentially improve consistency of data interpretation, the implementation of automated processes is desirable to generate standardized and structured data, supporting various downstream AI development projects that produce reliable models.

In 2021, 69 abstracts were accepted for publication, reporting either AI-based systems or sophisticated machine learning models with an impact on diagnosis, prognosis or therapeutic decision, a 40% increase on the previous two years. New AI-based models and prognostic systems with potential clinical impact are being developed at a rapid pace **[86]**.

### 2.3.1. Prognostic factors

These factors help physicians assess a patient's prognosis and make decisions about the best treatment approach. Using data such as that from flow cytometry analysis with AI, researchers were able to identify new prognostic factors in 56 pediatric patients with B-cell acute lymphoblastic leukemia (B-ALL) . Based on statistical correlation methods for relapse prediction, they identified differentiation cluster 38 (CD38 ) as a potential marker of relapse, indicating that B cells with low CD38 expression could serve as a potential indicator of relapse in patients with ALL **[87]**.

ML algorithms are part of a wider *"datamining"* approach to analyzing large, complex data sets, and are gradually finding their way into clinical practice. These techniques were applied to a retrospective Cohort in a European Society of Blood and Bone Marrow Transplantation registry study of 28,236 patients with acute leukemia, and enabled researchers to develop and validate a model to predict 100-day mortality after allogeneic hematopoietic stem cell transplantation. They used an interpretable model of boosted decision trees, taking into account variables such as patient age, disease score, and donor serological test results. The algorithm outperforms previous standards in outcome prediction for estimating overall mortality after allogeneic hematopoietic stem cell transplantation and evaluating its efficacy at two years **[88]**.

In hemostasis exploration, AI-based models have been used to predict thrombosis risk in patients with myeloproliferative neoplasms, demonstrating the ability of AI-based diagnostic support systems to improve diagnostic accuracy in hematology. Model input variables encompass patients' bioassay results, hemodynamic status and comorbidities to provide prediction of deep thrombosis risk up to 12 or 24 hours before the onset of associated symptoms, facilitating early management and prevention of complications **[46,89]**.

### 2.3.2. Risk scores

Disease risk scores are often used in clinical practice to help physicians assess a patient's individual risk and make decisions about disease prevention, screening and treatment. They can also be used in medical research to identify high-risk populations who could benefit from preventive interventions.

The *"Mutation-Enhanced International Prognostic Score System"* (MIPSS70), as a prognostic score for mortality in patients with primary myelofibrosis, is an example of a proportional hazards statistical model developed from data collected from 805 patients. By fitting the model to the data, the relationships between the variables and their impact on the outcome can be determined. However, creating the MIPSS70 involved deliberate choices on the part of the researchers. They had to decide which variables to include in the model. These variables can be specific patient characteristics, biological markers or other relevant factors. The variable selection process is often based on medical knowledge and a thorough understanding of the field **[90]**.

In addition, the researchers had to determine which variables were dependent and independent, i.e. which variables directly influenced the outcome and which were interconnected. They also examined possible interactions between variables, as certain combinations of factors may have a different impact on mortality **[90]**. The selected list of relevant variables included in the score questionnaire is illustrated in **figure 22**.

| # | Question | Answer |
|---|---|---|
| 1 | Severe Anemia (hemoglobin <80g/L) | ○ Yes ○ No |
| 2 | Moderate Anemia (hemoglobin 80-100g/L) | ○ Yes ○ No |
| 3 | Leucocytosis >25x10⁹/L | ○ Yes ○ No |
| 4 | Thrombocytopenia (platelet count <100x10⁹/L) | ○ Yes ○ No |
| 5 | Peripheral blood blast count ≥2% | ○ Yes ○ No |
| 6 | Bone marrow fibrosis grade ≥2 | ○ Yes ○ No |
| 7 | Constitutional symptoms | ○ Yes ○ No |
| 8 | Absence of CALR type 1/like mutation | ○ Yes ○ No |
| 9 | HMR[1] category | ○ Yes ○ No |
| 10 | ≥2 HMR mutated genes | ○ Yes ○ No |
| 11 | Unfavorable karyotype[2] | ○ Yes ○ No ○ Not available |
| 12 | Very High Risk karyotype[3] | ○ Yes ○ No ○ Not available |
| | **Score** | **Result** |
| | MIPSS70 | |
| | MIPSS70-plus version 2.0 | |

**Figure 22 MIPSS70 and MIPSS70-plus score form: questions include mortality-related variables [91]**

***CALR:*** *"Calreticulin*

***HMR:*** *Hight Molecular Risk*

Another highly promising study tackled the complex problem of diagnosing disseminated intravascular coagulation (DIC). Currently, the diagnosis of DIC is tedious and involves the interpretation of a combination of laboratory and clinical parameters through the use of certain probability scores. In this study, the authors used a supervised neural network model analyzing 32 clinical and laboratory parameters in an initial development model on 656 suspected DIC patients (428 healthy and 228 with confirmed DIC) and subsequently in an external validation model on 217 patients (137 healthy and 80 with DIC) and compared its diagnostic performance with that of three widely used probability scores (International Society of Thrombosis and

Hemostasis, Japanese Ministry of Health and Welfare, and Japanese Association of Acute Medicine). Not only did the ML model outperform the three scores, but it also revealed that certain variables generally overlooked for the diagnosis of DIC, such as the number of eosinophils in the blood or the distribution width of platelets or red blood cells, are of some importance in the diagnosis of DIC **[92]**.

Another widely explored area with very encouraging results is that of predicting the risk of venous thromboembolism (VTE) or its recurrence in different patient populations. An interesting example is the identification of high-risk VTE subjects among medically ill patients. Currently, prediction is based on clinical scores, such as the Padua scores or *the International Medical Prevention Registry on Venous Thromboembolism* (IMPROVE), which, however, have little predictive value. The application of two ML algorithms using supervised learning, analyzing respectively 68 and 16 variables from 7513 patients enrolled in the APEX clinical trial, showed that these two AI systems significantly outperformed the IMPROVE score in the prediction of VTE **[93,94]**. Combining regression model estimates and ML techniques, these algorithms encompass previously unused risk factors and provide a qualitatively better calibrated score than traditional methods **[93]**.

### 2.3.3. Predictive biomarkers

Predictive biomarkers in hematology, aided by AI methods, are revolutionizing the way blood-related diseases are diagnosed and treated.

Some recent examples of the use of supervised learning in the field of hemostasis have involved some commonly used coagulation biomarkers, such as the D-dimer assay. In a study carried out by Wang at Zhengzhou University in China **[95]**a supervised learning model was able to determine which biomarker can better differentiate patients with thrombotic thrombocytopenic purpura who are at risk of adverse outcomes. In this study, the AI model was used to establish that admission D-dimer had the best prognostic value **[96]**.

Another controversial diagnostic issue is that of heparin-induced thrombocytopenia (HIT), which also involves the combined interpretation of clinical parameters and biological biomarkers. By implementing these parameters in various algorithms proposed in a prospective multicenter cohort study including 1393 patients suspected of HIT, a supervised ML model applied to a subset of training data (75% of patients) and a validation data set (25% of patients) was significantly more accurate in diagnosing HIT than currently recommended algorithms **[92]**.

### 2.3.4. Disease staging

The staging of haemopathies, such as blood cancers (leukemias, lymphomas, myelomas, etc.) and haematological disorders (anaemias, thrombocytopenia, etc.), is a crucial process for assessing the extent of the disease and guiding therapeutic management.

According to the *"French American British"* (FAB) classification of , leukemia is classified into two main types: lymphoblastic and myeloid, with specific subtypes. Diagnosis of acute lymphoblastic leukemia is often guided by a comprehensive blood test, then requires bone marrow aspiration and microscopic examination of the bone marrow smear for confirmation. Computer-assisted diagnostic methods have become more efficient and accurate than manual methods, offering new opportunities to improve leukemia detection **[97]**. However, challenges remain, particularly in the classification of acute lymphoblastic leukemia subtypes, due to their variability and similarity. Accurate diagnosis is of crucial importance in determining the optimal treatment plan for each patient. A pre-trained CNN,

AlexNet, has been shown to classify ALL into 3 types on the basis of blood smears, with a specificity of 99.03%. Without having to go through the first step of segmenting microscopic images, or using the *"K-means"* and *"fuzzy C-means"* techniques for *"clustering"* used in previous work for the classification of leukemias, the AlexNet automated model stands out with superior performance indicators and promises accurate diagnosis for early management **[98]**. The three types of fully interconnected CNN layers are represented in **Figure 23** by three distinct colors and classify cells into: Normal, Type L1, L2 or L3.

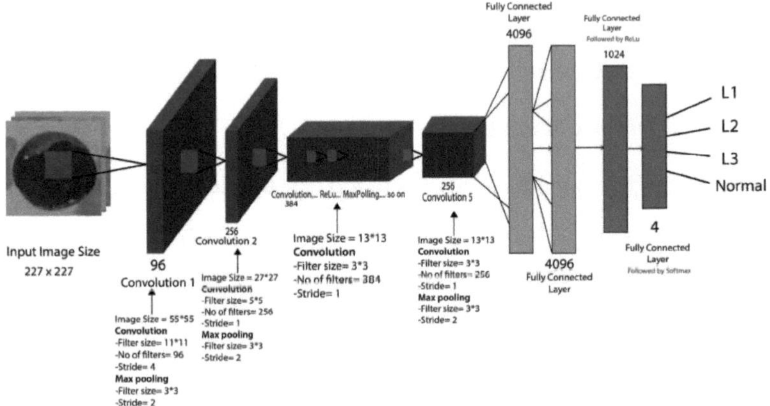


**Figure 23 :Architecture of the AlexNet network for the classification of acute lymphocytic leukemias [98]**

Another research work presented in 2018 a complete architecture based on deep learning techniques to classify LALs achieving 97.78% accuracy with efficient processing time. The system includes convolution and *"max-pooling"* layers to train the model, as well as fully connected layers to classify the image. This time, the approach segments the bone marrow image and classifies it as normal or as leukemic belonging to one of the subtypes L1, L2 and L3 depending on the marrow assignment. The convolutional neural network is used to understand deep features and improve the classification accuracy of the trained model, providing a valuable disease staging tool for laboratory experts and pathologists, which is crucial for leukemia patients **[99]**.

## 2.4. Clinical decision support systems

The integration of AI into clinical decision-making is based on recent advances in machine learning and data analysis. These systems harness big data to support clinicians in diagnosis, treatment option selection and outcome prediction. Using machine learning techniques, they identify complex patterns in the data, improving the accuracy of treatment recommendations and healthcare management. A presented model integrates medical guidelines, latest practices, expert knowledge and ML algorithms to reveal correlations between patient profiles, treatment protocols and predicted outcomes. Given the lack of relevant data in the historical files needed to train the system, a computer program capable of generating infinite virtual scenarios reflecting the distribution of disease in the population was developed. It works by capturing all the important factors concerning the anonymous clinical profile of the patient receiving treatment for chronic lymphocytic leukemia (CLL) and then produces a detailed report concerning treatment alternatives. The report presents all the factors influencing the decision and their relative impacts **[100]**.

Supervised learning is the most commonly used technique for building clinical models that can aid hematologists in diagnosis, prognosis or therapeutic decisions. This approach focuses on classifications and requires carefully organized datasets with labeled observations to learn a function that maps input data (e.g. images of different cells) to the desired output (e.g. classification of cell types) based on the input-output pairs provided (e.g.

labeled images). Training the model iteratively refines its performance, aligning predictions with labeled data. Model accuracy is assessed by evaluating its performance on a selected data set **[101]**.

Accurate screening for iron-deficiency anemia, reticulocytosis, hereditary spherocytosis and diabetes is possible using a machine-learning model. This CNN predicts pathophysiological conditions from the analysis of red blood cells, using their cellular morphological, chemical and mechanical properties. These properties are fed into the neural network as an input vector to provide output data corresponding to the predicted diagnosis, with an accuracy of 98%. The proposed method enables rapid and efficient screening of multiple diseases and syndromes compared with conventional methods, by exploiting the performance of machine learning models **[102]**.

## 2.5. Personalized medicine: Optimizing treatments and therapeutic protocols in hematology

A more sophisticated technique is reinforcement learning (RL), which has become quite popular but has been relatively untested in healthcare, let alone hematology. In RL, an agent performs various operations to interact with an environment with the aim of maximizing its expected gain, similar to situations where clinicians need to adjust their action (treatment) according to a patient's conditions (e.g. genetic profile). Thus, RL could be used to optimize the treatment of patients with distinct characteristics, and model performance can be further improved by effectively combining RL with DL **[103]**.

Many decision-making problems in medicine are intrinsically sequential. When a patient consults a doctor, the latter must decide what treatment to administer. When the patient returns, the previously administered treatment influences his or her current state and, consequently, the next decision concerning future treatment. This type of decision problem can be efficiently modeled and solved using RL algorithms. Unlike most AI systems implemented in medicine, which ignore the sequential nature of decisions, RL offers an attractive alternative by taking into account not only the immediate effect of treatment, but also the long-term benefit to the patient. However, the application of RL algorithms in the hospital presents obstacles, as these algorithms generally learn by trial and error, which is not a practical option for exploratory treatments on patients. A crucial issue is also determining the reward, which influences optimal policy behavior. Despite these challenges, there are examples of successful applications of RL in medicine, notably to develop treatment strategies for epilepsy, lung cancer, and sepsis. In the field of nephrology, the treatment of anemia in hemodialysis patients lends itself well to modeling as a sequential decision problem, where RL can be used to guide the administration of erythropoiesis-stimulating agents **[103]**.

The researchers also applied an unsupervised learning technique for hierarchical clustering on gene expression data. This method makes it possible to group similar data into clusters without having pre-labels on the data. In this case, gene expression data were collected from patients with diffuse large B-cell lymphoma. The results of this hierarchical clustering showed that lymphoma could be grouped into two main motifs: the germinal center and the activated B cell. These patterns probably reflect specific molecular characteristics of the tumors. These classifications were then associated with the prediction of response to treatment. In other words, the subtypes identified by the hierarchical classification correlated with how well patients responded to treatment, suggesting that gene expression-based classification can provide useful information for predicting the efficacy of therapies in diffuse large B-cell lymphoma. This highlights the importance of molecular data analysis for a thorough understanding of disease subtypes and their responses to treatment **[104]**.

Currently, *"IBM Watson for Oncology"* uses machine learning algorithms and natural language processing of the electronic medical record to combine patient and disease characteristics, published literature, available clinical trials and oncologists' experience to suggest and rank treatment options **[101,105]**

By analyzing genetic and molecular data, AI can predict how a patient will respond to a particular treatment. For example, for lymphoma patients, AI models can help determine which therapies will be most effective for specific genetic profiles. This has made it possible to exploit multidimensional oncology data to predict, for example, the efficacy of immune checkpoint inhibitors, which are monoclonal immunotherapy antibodies used in the treatment of certain cancers **[105]**.

### 2.6. Improved management of medical data and electronic records

With the massive increase in healthcare data generated by biological analyses, electronic medical records and medical imaging systems, AI can help healthcare professionals better exploit *"Big Data"* and manage the flow of this valuable information.

As part of a project to prioritize hospital stays, a management tool based on an algorithm for assigning a score to each hospital stay has been designed using the Groupe Hospitalier Paris Saint-Joseph's databases, to help prioritize the reasons for stays and improve hospitalization pricing, particularly in the case of diseases of the blood and hematopoietic organs. The model takes into account patient history and disease severity for the 10150 re-evaluated stays, in order to estimate the length of stay required and the means of management that will subsequently be applied to similar scenarios. **[106]**.

Another tool already in place in Boston, this time included 2,997,249 cases of hospitalization lasting more than 21 days, to enable the development of an algorithm for predicting the length of stay of future patients using a regression method. This advance is based on the exploitation of data from 2014 to 2021, to set up this predictive model for emergency departments, which subsequently inspired several hospital groups in **Europe [107].**

Medical information can sometimes seem complex to patients, and AI has become an essential resource for understanding their own state of health. This can be achieved thanks to a tool developed by "*Vital*" that translates complex medical terms from hospital databases into simple, understandable language. The model uses previously collected data such as laboratory results or doctor's notes and couples them with NLP techniques to improve comprehension, reducing the workload and time spent explaining diagnoses and treatments **[108,109]**.

# 3. ADVANTAGES AND LIMITATIONS OF USING ARTIFICIAL INTELLIGENCE IN HEMATOLOGY

AI is improving the quality of healthcare, and its increasing integration into tomorrow's medicine is opening up promising new prospects, particularly for the diagnosis of blood diseases and decision-making in associated conditions. However, it is crucial to emphasize that this technology, which must be used in the interests of both doctors and patients, must be rigorously regulated to avoid any potential pitfalls.

## 3.1. The potential impact of artificial intelligence in hematology

Technological advances promise significant breakthroughs in several key areas of hematology, including oncohaematology, hematopoietic stem cell development and infection detection.

### 3.1.1. Oncohaematology

AI has recently changed the panorama of oncology investigation through the use of machine learning algorithms. Studies based on DL as well as ML propose future strategies to challenge these negative prognostic pathologies via in-depth omic analysis, detection of new markers and classification accuracy for optimal therapy selection and better assessment of relapse and survival **[110]**.

#### 3.1.1.1. In-depth multi-omics analysis

Oncology relies on evidence-based evaluation systems for the diagnosis, staging and treatment of cancer. These systems have developed with the introduction of more advanced tests such as next-generation genetic sequencing. This has led to a growing list of prognostic and predictive factors, but their complexity makes them difficult to understand with traditional approaches. AI offers a solution by exploiting ML and DL algorithms to analyze multimodal data and identify complex patterns **(Figure 24) [111]**.

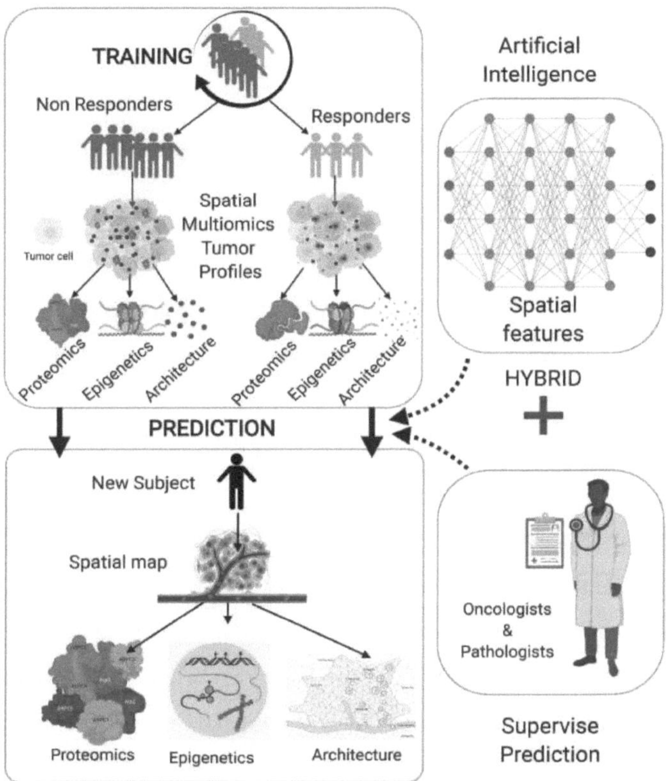


**Figure 24Precision diagnostics in oncology by integrating artificial intelligence into multi-omics analyses. [112]**

Samples and biopsies are analyzed to characterize tumor compositions. As shown in **figure 24**, AI uses this data to predict personalized treatment plans, supervised by experts. Next-generation clinical trials will validate personalized therapies **[112]**.

An emerging strategy for cancer screening is the development of a *"Pan-Cancer Atlas"* based on blood sequencing. It can also be used to deduce the phenotypic and functional characteristics of *"Natural Killer"* (NK) cell clusters in each type of cancer. Indeed, transcription factor regulation and cell communication prediction algorithms have been applied to understand the mechanisms of NK cell populations within tumors and their strategies for combating tumor cells **[113]**. These algorithms enable precise analysis of genomic and transcriptomic data, offering promising prospects for early detection, cancer classification and prediction of response to treatment.

#### 3.1.1.2. Biomarkers

Recent advances in molecular analysis techniques, such as multiparametric flow cytometry, mass spectrometry and genomic sequencing, have enabled the identification of new biomarkers and improved our understanding of the underlying mechanisms of blood cancers.

Two other conventional methods for studying biomarkers in the tumor microenvironment have been greatly enhanced by AI, i.e. immunofluorescence (IF) and immunohistochemistry (IHC ). They enable biomarker measurements using sets of antibodies conjugated to distinct spectral fluorochromes. Although they have been used in many clinical and research projects, achieving multiplex IF and IHC is still crucial for more data-driven cellular research in immunology and cancer biology. To address this, AI algorithms have developed optimized tools for profiling a panel of over 24 biomarkers in cancer patient cells using IF and IHC techniques. These protein imaging methods are early efforts in a computational view of proteomic biomarkers that is impacting next-generation oncology analysis **[112]**.

On the other hand, oncohaematology researchers and AI experts conducted a multicenter cohort study in 3 hospital centers in the USA in 2019 to highlight the importance of machine learning technologies in translating genomic biomarker data into useful clinical tools. Studying the contribution of biomarkers in predicting resistance to DNA methylation inhibiting agents in patients with myelodysplastic syndromes identified, with high accuracy, the probability of having resistance to this chemotherapy **[114]**.

#### 3.1.1.3. Classification aid

In the microscopic analysis of blood cells, particularly in the context of lymphomas and leukemias, there may be slight morphological variations between different classes of cells. These differences may be difficult to discern with the naked eye, and may not be evident on standard examination. However, these morphological subtleties can have important diagnostic significance in specifically identifying the cell type and nature of the disease. Based on blood test data, two merged CNNs promise to provide the correct diagnostic prediction of all patients with promyelocytic leukemia and myeloid leukemia. Sensitivity, specificity and accuracy values of 100%, 92.3% and 93.7%, respectively, were achieved for myeloid leukemia. For lymphoid leukemia, a sensitivity of 89% and specificity and accuracy values of 100% were obtained. This model has been shown to distinguish neoplastic diseases (leukemia) from non-neoplastic diseases (infections) and also to recognize the leukemic lineage **[115]**.

Another major diagnostic challenge in characterizing morphological variants of peripheral blood elements is the detection of dysplasia. Identification of these abnormalities is essential for the diagnosis of myelodysplastic syndromes and other associated disorders.

The cytoplasmic hypogranularity of neutrophils associated with myelodysplastic syndrome may present high rates of interobserver variability. LD-based predictions could provide additional objective tools to address this issue. *"DysplasiaNet"* is a CNN model that has been designed and trained for automatic recognition of cytoplasmic hypogranularity in dysplastic neutrophils. This LD model will be able to identify them consistently from digital blood smear images. The resulting cell images undergo dimensionality reduction using the t-SNE technique to give two polynuclear clusters: normal or dysplastic **[116]**.

### 3.1.1. Hematopoietic stem cells

One of the current challenges in studies of human physiological mechanisms and associated pathologies is the lack of models that accurately reproduce the complex functions of human organs. The demand for experiments on human organ models in place of animal validation studies is a proposal emerging as part of efforts to reduce, replace and refine (the 3Rs) the use of animals in biomedical research. Devices that recreate the cellular microenvironments of specific human organs, enabling cellular interactions, drug responses and disease mechanisms to be studied in a more precise and relevant way than traditional animal models. Technological advances have enabled scientists to better replicate the human cell microenvironment using bioreactors that maintain certain properties of hematopoietic stem cells (HSCs) **[117]**.

Understanding the mechanisms regulating HSCs opens the way to new potential applications of AI in modeling the complex molecular networks that control HSC fate, in order to identify new therapeutic targets or optimize in vitro differentiation protocols.

#### 3.1.1.1. Bone marrow in three dimensions

Recent advances have made it possible to generate an in vitro protocol for obtaining a minimalist, standardized system that is easy to set up and offers features of a bone marrow-like structure, combining different cell populations, reflecting the heterogeneity of medullary tissue in vivo. This three-dimensional (3D) bone marrow-like structure, assembled using calcium phosphate-based particles and human cell lines representative of the bone marrow microenvironment, enables a wide variety of biological processes to be monitored by combining or replacing different primary cell populations within the system. The final 3D structures can then be harvested for computer imaging analysis **[118]**. From this 3D model, it is possible to replace each cell type with primary cells, normal or pathological, or even add other cell types to enhance biomimetic properties, such as immune cells, adipocytes or fibroblasts. The addition of other cell types could facilitate studies of other problems, such as the extent of local bone marrow inflammation or resistance to immunotherapy **[118]**.

#### 3.1.1.2. *Ex-vivo* hematopoiesis

The study of hematopoiesis, whether normal or pathological, is complex and requires a multidisciplinary approach. Mathematical models have been developed to understand cell dynamics, cancer development and treatment efficacy. Using these models, calibrated on the basis of experimental data, it is possible to study the complete process of hematopoiesis. Modeling altered hematopoiesis, particularly in the case of blood cancers, can reveal the cell types involved in dysfunction, offering therapeutic leads. Although the biology of cancer cells is more complex than that of models, the latter focus on the key parameters influencing the dynamics of hematological malignancies, making it possible to highlight the characteristics of mutated cells that could be targeted by therapies to restore normal hematopoiesis **[119]**.

On the other hand, aging of the bone marrow microenvironment has been shown to contribute critically to the decline in HSC function over time.

Paradoxically, while some BM structures degrade with age and negatively affect HSC function, other specific cells and signals are preserved to maintain HSC function and regenerative capacity. Of note, an exponential impact in the understanding of this biological system has recently been made by single-cell genomic sequencing techniques, spatial transcriptomics, and the implementation of artificial intelligence and DL approaches to data analysis and integration. For example, the development of co-culture systems mimicking OM *ex vivo*, highlights the importance of new technologies in elucidating the complexity of its aging mechanism **[120]**.

### 3.1.2. Hematological diagnosis of infections

An example of a revolutionary tool in the detection of hematological infections has been designed to rapidly screen a thick smear slide for parasites. It's a DL application for smartphones capable of detecting malaria parasites coupled with a CNN model. The system involves a smartphone taking an image of the blood smear through the microscope lens, and the app analyzing it. Detection accuracy is estimated at 97.26%, with very high specificity and sensitivity. This is explained by the AUC, which approaches one in **figure 25**, testifying to the high performance of the model. **[121]**.

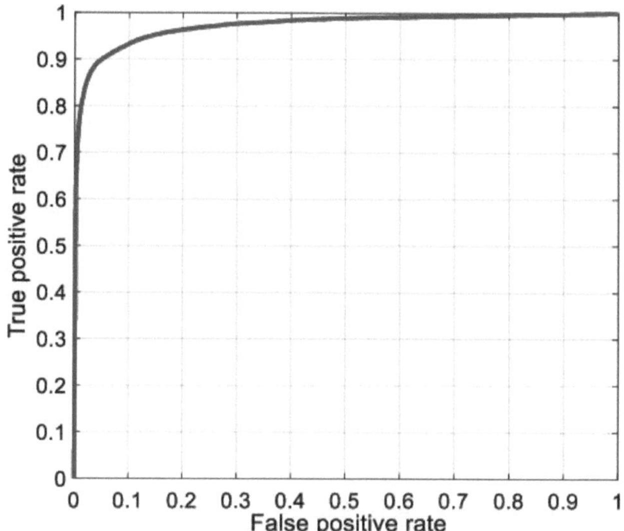


**Figure 25Sensitivity versus specificity curve of the system for detecting malaria-infected erythrocytes from a thick smear using a mobile application. [121]**

Another machine learning tool developed in January 2024 by researchers at the Laboratoire de biologie des microorganismes et biotechnologie in Oran and the École nationale d'électronique et des télécommunications in Sfax used a linear regression model to detect pulmonary and extra-pulmonary tuberculosis based on blood counts and socio-demographic data. This will make it possible to create diagnostic methods that are both highly effective and economical, especially given that the countries most affected are those with low incomes **[122]**.

### 3.2.Outlook and future developments

Although the human brain is extremely powerful, it has limitations in terms of information processing capacity and memory, compared with a computer. AI therefore plays a crucial role in supporting human intelligence to produce reliable results, enabling faster, more accurate diagnoses and better patient care. What's more, AI offers promising prospects in the processing of large quantities of data, which is essential for scientific progress by enabling researchers to make faster progress in understanding the development of diseases, diagnosis, the personalization of treatments, and even the prediction and prevention of certain pathologies **[123]**.

### 3.2.1. Bioanalyzer performance

The interrelation between AI and biological analysis instruments is very close in medical bioengineering. These instruments generate a wide variety of complex data, such as spectral, mass spectrometric and electrochemical data. AI algorithms enable these data to be processed, identifying trends, characteristics and differences between samples. They also facilitate pattern recognition and classification of analytical instruments to diagnose analyzer capabilities by monitoring performance data and proposing usage recommendations **[17]**.

This synergy between AI and analysis tools enables data consolidation and global analysis, helping researchers to optimize the performance of bioanalyzers and increase their fields of use.

The AU5800 Automatic Biochemical Analyzer is an advanced example. Widely used to perform many types of routine biochemical tests, researchers suggest that it may be possible to extend its uses in hematology to reflect the degree of hemolysis of red blood cells, through a complete analysis of the biological constants involved. In addition, it may be able to monitor analysis results in real time, identifying abnormal conditions and taking automatic action. This will improve the efficiency of laboratory analysis and the accuracy of results, help identify potential disease risk factors, and predict disease development in advance, facilitating early intervention and diagnosis in the case of hemolytic syndrome **[124]**.

A new methodology that combines the use of a microfluidic unit with machine-learning data analysis from video-recorded images will enable the assessment of red blood cell plasticity abnormalities in patients with rare hereditary hemolytic anemia. This technique promises to differentiate sickle cell disease, thalassemia and hereditary spherocytosis through improved characterization of red blood cells in autoimmune hemolytic anemia, which will allow patients to be stratified according to severity and/or response to treatment **[125]**.

### 3.2.2. The promise of precision medicine

Clearly, AI-based models will not replace hematologists in diagnosis and therapy selection, but rather assist them and free them from redundant and time-consuming tasks. This will enable hematologists to focus on complex cases and tasks requiring unique human skills.

In biomedicine, the aim is to remain at the forefront of this trend, as forecasts for 2025 suggest, placing the medical field as the one experiencing the strongest data growth. This mainly encompasses three types of data detailed in **Table VI [126]**.

**Table VIDescriptions and benefits of different types of medical data [126]**

| Data type | Description |
|---|---|
| **Genomic data** | Gene banks: A collection of genetic sequences stored for research or analysis. |
| | Genomes: complete sequences of an individual's genetic material, which can be used for omics studies. |
| **Biometric data** | Cardiovascular and metabolic parameters<br>Control of organic functions (kidney, liver, thyroid)<br>Blood count and hemodynamic parameters |
| **Clinical data** | Medical history<br>Laboratory test results<br>X-ray images: |

This abundance of information has transformed the way experiments are conducted, moving from small to large populations, generating more results requiring holistic analysis **[126]**.

Thanks to advances in AI, notably the use of artificial neural networks and supervised or unsupervised learning approaches, it is possible to integrate and analyze these vast datasets efficiently. This analysis makes it possible to stratify patients into homogeneous subgroups, called endotypes, based on underlying pathophysiological mechanisms. This stratification offers prospects for precision medicine, where treatments can be tailored according to the specific characteristics of each patient subgroup **[127].**

### 3.2.3. Discovering new therapeutic avenues

Another important application of disease modeling is the identification of potential therapeutic targets. By analyzing molecular data through modeling, researchers can identify genes or proteins that play a central role in regulating biological systems disrupted by pathology. These identified molecules constitute promising therapeutic targets for the development of new drugs **[127].**

Advanced computational analyses have been used to identify and optimize potential drugs that can specifically target the identified therapeutic targets. Sophisticated algorithms are used to select the most promising chemical molecules or biological compounds, then optimize them to improve their pharmacological properties **[128].**

AI also facilitates the design, implementation and monitoring of clinical studies evaluating new drugs. It enables better selection of patients and study sites, as well as advanced analyses of data generated during clinical studies and in silico drug evaluation. Clinical trial simulations based on AI models offer promising prospects for reducing the costs and time associated with clinical trials, while improving their design and probability of success **(Figure 26) [127].**

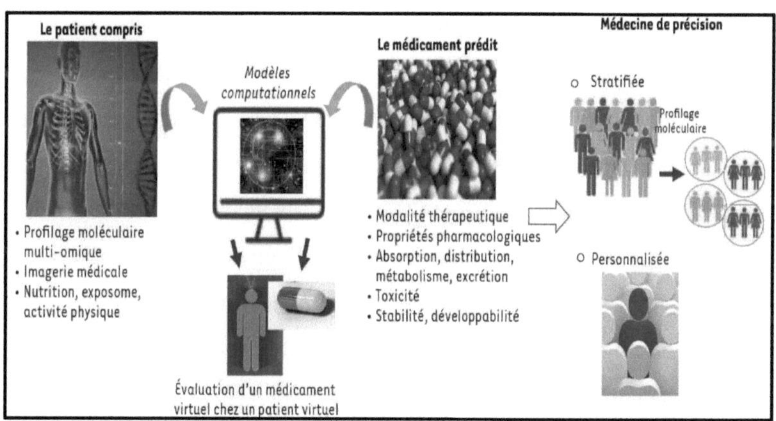


**Figure 26:Computational artificial intelligence and the prediction of precision treatment regimens [127]**

### 3.3.The ethical and scientific challenges of artificial intelligence

In medical settings, AI integration increases diagnostic accuracy, reduces overall healthcare costs, facilitates information sharing and improves targeted treatments. However, the development of AI systems in clinical practice presents a unique set of challenges that must be addressed to ensure their accuracy and reliability.

AI in the medical field is hoped for its ability to detect complex problems quickly, thus promoting preventive medicine. However, its growing adoption raises ethical and legal concerns, particularly with regard to patient consent to the use of their data, the responsibility of healthcare professionals in dealing with AI, and the implications of its predictions on the patient's state of health. However, the use of this powerful technology must be justified by its benefit to caregivers and patients, and its development and use must be strictly regulated to avoid abuses **[123]**.

### 3.3.1. Technical flaws and reliability of results

A recent study involving 457 clinicians across 13 US states explored their diagnostic performance when asked to respond to a clinical vignette related to respiratory distress, either without assistance or with the support of an AI system for interpreting chest radiographs. The study showed that diagnostic performance was slightly improved by AI assistance, but also, worryingly, that when the AI system was biased, diagnostic performance was significantly deteriorated. Therefore, even for healthcare professionals, AI support for complex clinical case diagnosis and decision-making should be adopted with caution, strictly monitoring system performance **[92]**.

Despite the promising results obtained with the complex architectures of artificial neural networks, several challenges remain to be solved for the clinical application of deep learning to healthcare.

#### 3.3.1.1. Data volume

DL refers to a set of highly intensive computational models. A typical example is that of fully connected *"multilayer"* neural networks, where many network parameters need to be estimated correctly. The basis for achieving this goal is the availability of a huge amount of data. However, healthcare is a different domain, with around 7.5 billion people in the world (as of September 2016), a large proportion of whom have no access to primary healthcare **[129]**. Consequently, we can't get as many patients as we'd like to train a targeted comprehensive deep learning model. Furthermore, understanding diseases and their variability is much more complicated than for other tasks, such as image or speech recognition. As a result, from a megadata perspective, the amount of medical data required to train an effective and robust deep learning model would be much greater compared with other media **[129].**

#### 3.3.1.2. Data quality

Unlike other domains where data is clean and well-structured, healthcare data is highly heterogeneous, ambiguous and incomplete. Training a good DL model with such massive and varied datasets is challenging and requires taking into account several issues, such as data sparsity, redundancy and missing values. Consequently, it is essential to ensure that the data used to train AI algorithms are of high quality, free from bias, and include variations among patient histories and **clinical** conditions **[130]**. On the other hand, in certain situations where the incidence of hematological diseases is rare, representative information may not be able to be acquired to develop AI-based models for prediction, diagnosis and risk stratification. A possible example would be the lymphoma *"Mucosa-associated lymphoid tissue"* (MALT) and other lymphomas such as enteropathic T lymphoma. In such conditions, AI fails due to its inability to obtain the global solution to the problem and tends to remain limited due to the size and quality of the data **[130].**

#### 3.3.1.3. Temporality

Diseases always progress and evolve over time in unpredictable ways. However, many existing deep learning models, including those already proposed in the medical field, assume inputs based on static vectors, which cannot handle the time factor in a natural way. Designing deep learning approaches capable of handling temporal health variations is an important aspect that will require the development of innovative solutions **[129].**

#### 3.3.1.4. Interpretability

Although LD models have been successful in many application areas, they are often compared to black boxes whose operating details are not elucidated. However, in healthcare, not only is quantitative algorithmic performance important, but also the reasoning behind the algorithms is relevant. In fact, such interpretability of the model (i.e. providing which phenotypes influence the predictions, for example) is crucial in convincing healthcare professionals of the actions recommended by the predictive system (e.g. prescription of a specific drug, potential high risk of developing a certain disease) **[129]**.

In some cases, the source data used to develop a model may present significant intra-observer or intra-institutional variability, making it difficult to establish a reliable reference for assessing model performance. In such situations, the absence of a reliable reference standard limits the reliability of the model **[131].**

What's more, most machine learning-based studies are carried out on datasets from a single institution, which is a major potential limitation on their generalizability. "*Watson for Oncology*", a project by *International Business Machines Corporation* developed as a support system for oncologists, is a striking example. Although *"Watson for Oncology"* can integrate multiple sources of information (electronic medical record data and oncology literature) into its decisions, studies of its clinical use have noted limitations in its ability to adapt its recommendations to local practices, older patients and medically complex or ambiguous cases **[132]**. This example highlights the importance of taking care to consider the outcome data used to train a model, as well as the challenge associated with deploying a model in new environments.

The lack of interpretability in predictive ML models should prompt caution, especially when the decisions made may have an impact on patients' health and lives. Indeed, AI models more often than not lack the broader clinical context that is relevant to patient care **[92]**.

### 3.3.2. Ethical issues: Decision-making and the threat to fairness

To develop responsible and ethical AI, it is essential to prioritize the needs of doctors and patients. Economic pressure must never dictate the development and use of AI models. **[123]**.

However, it is essential to stress that the use of these technologies must be accompanied by ethical vigilance and consideration of data confidentiality issues, thus ensuring that these advances benefit both individuals and society as a whole.

As data becomes increasingly detailed and the need to share data between institutions becomes apparent, patients' privacy and data rights must also be taken into account. Even for supposedly de-identified data, there is a concern that personal information could potentially be inferred from publicly available LD models, exposing a conflict between the desire to make machine learning useful to the medical community as a whole and the need to protect the privacy of patients who contribute to research efforts. Furthermore, for datasets containing highly detailed genomic information, the question arises as to whether true anonymization is possible; patient consent is then essential to guarantee medical ethics **[129].**

If AI is to be at the service of patients, data management must be rigorously regulated to avoid any abuses in its use. The Commission Nationale de l'Informatique et des Libertés (CNIL), in a 2017 report, highlighted two founding principles for the use of AI in medical settings, stressing that the interests of users must take precedence over all other considerations **[133].** The first principle is that of the fairness of algorithms, which must be loyal to users as citizens and not just as consumers, taking into account collective and not just individual impacts. The second principle is that of vigilance, which implies regular, deliberative evaluation of algorithms, involving all stakeholders via ethics committees. To put these principles into practice, the report stipulates the need for ethics training for all players in the algorithmic chain, and for greater transparency of systems within companies via ethics committees **[133].**

### 3.3.3. Legal issues for healthcare applications

Potential errors or abuses of AI in medicine are prompting a call for rigorous regulations, from both scientific societies and government authorities. These regulations aim to ensure continuous monitoring, combining integrated mechanisms for rapid regulatory updates, to guide the ongoing progress of AI capabilities in medicine and science. Indeed, President Biden issued a Presidential Executive Order on the implications of AI for healthcare organizations on October 30, 2023, urging agencies to establish standards for the safe and reliable use of AI **[123]**. In addition, the European Union has developed rules for AI use that will soon be adopted, and the World Health Organization has published a detailed document on regulatory considerations for AI use in healthcare **[134].** Careful monitoring of the evolving implications of AI use in healthcare and research, with the establishment of limits to prevent abuse, and balancing awareness of the considerable benefits and advances that AI can bring, seems to be the best approach for framing the application of this revolutionary technology in the medical field, without stifling its innovative and beneficial potential **[92]**.

The European Commission is currently debating the question of granting robots legal personality, as existing texts, such as the directive on product liability for defective products number 85/374/EEC, **[135]** are not adapted to the evolution of AI.

Advocates of strict regulation suggest a process similar to the controls applied when marketing medical devices or drugs. They argue that without extreme scientific rigor, the risk of exposing patients to potentially fatal errors would be too high **[123]**.

The future challenge will probably be human supervision of AI developments, what Dr. D. Gruzon calls "the human guarantee". This translates into human supervision of any use of digital technology in healthcare involving three main actors; the patient who must be informed of any act based on AI algorithms, healthcare professionals who master the limits and uses of these systems and AI designers who ensure the explicability of models **[136].**

# CONCLUSION

The growing integration of AI in medicine in general, and in hematology in particular, is paving the way for a profound transformation in medical practices, with potential benefits including reduced diagnostic times and costs, as well as prediction of specific pathologies and treatments.

The use of these innovative technologies in hematology laboratories offers the promise of standardization, improved process efficiency and reduced staff workload for repetitive, automatable tasks. This frees up valuable resources that can be reallocated to more important activities such as patient care, research and development, and continuous process improvement.

However, it cannot totally replace healthcare professionals due to its limitations, such as limited databases, the risk of errors and the need for rigorous clinical validation. It is imperative that all players (researchers, practitioners and patients) approach these challenges with caution and ethics, in order to maximize benefits while minimizing risks. To this end, specific, strict regulations are needed to govern its use in medicine, and to guarantee the reliability of results and respect for confidentiality. To make progress in this field, more research is needed, and AI must be integrated into the medical training of clinicians and healthcare professionals.

The future of hematology will be profoundly influenced by AI. By continuing to explore and exploit the possibilities offered by this technology, it is possible to significantly improve patient care, advance medical research and open up new vistas for innovation in the medical field.

# REFERENCES


1. Obstfeld AE. Hematology and machine learning. J Appl Lab Med. 2023;8(1):129-44.
2. Bajwa J, Munir U, Nori A, Williams B. Artificial intelligence in healthcare: Transforming the practice of medicine. Future Healthc J. 2021;8(2):188-94.
3. Charles YP, Lamas V, Ntilikina Y. Artificial intelligence and treatment algorithms in spinal surgery. Rev Chir Orthop Traumatol. 2022;108(6):147-55.
4. De Sousa Cardoso C, Galou E, Kervella A, KwoK P. Data power: Understand and harness the value of data. Paris: Eyrolles; 2020.
5. Brunelle F, Brunelle P. Artificial intelligence and medical imaging: definition, state of the art and perspectives. Bull Acad Natl Med. 2019;203(8):683-7.
6. Jean A. A brief introduction to artificial intelligence. Med Sci. 2020;36(11):1059-67.
7. Ascoli S. Understanding the artificial intelligence revolution. Paris : Editions First; 2020.
8. Janiesch C, Zschech P, Heinrich K. Machine learning and deep learning. Electron Mark. 2021;31(3):685-95.
9. Alassadi A, Ivanauskas T. Classification performance between machine learning and traditional programming in java [Thesis]. Kristianstad, Sweden: Faculty of Natural Sciences; 2019.
10. Chrisley R, Begeer S. Artificial intelligence: Critical concepts. United Kingdom: Taylor & Francis; 2000.

11. Touzet C. Artificial neural networks, introduction to connectionism [Online]. 2016 [Accessed 02/06/2024]. Available at: https://amu.hal.science/hal-01338010/document
12. Tano AJ. Automated translation of African languages. Cas du lingala [Master in Data Science]. Cote D'ivoire: Ministère de l'Enseignement Supérieur et de la Recherche Scientifique; 2020.
13. Xu M, Jin J, Wang G, Segers AJ, Deng T, Lin H. Machine learning based bias correction for numerical chemical transport models. Atmos Environ. 2021;248:118022.
14. Kimura K, Tabe Y, Ai T, Takehara I, Fukuda H, Takahashi H, et al. A novel automated image analysis system using deep convolutional neural networks can assist to differentiate MDS and AA. Sci Rep. 2019;9:13385.
15. Botros J, Mourad-Chehade F, Laplanche D. Automatic stratification of heart failure using a convolutional neural network. In: Colloque en TéléSANté et dispositifs biomédicaux, Université Paris 8, CNRS" Jun 2023, Paris Saint Denis, France. ffhal-04220664f
16. Li Y, Su H, Qi CR, Fish N, Cohen-Or D, Guibas LJ. Joint embeddings of shapes and images via CNN image purification. ACM Trans Graph. 2015;34(6):1-12.
17. Gavas E, Olpadkar K. Deep CNNs for Peripheral Blood Cell Classification [Preprint]. arXiv; 2021. https://doi.org/10.48550/arXiv.1909.09586
18. Poitier P. Automatic segmentation of sign language from French-speaking Belgium using recurrent neural networks [Dissertation]. Brussels: Université de Namur; 2022.
19. Balcerac A, Tervil B, Vayatis N, Ricard D. Fundamentals of machine learning for neurologists. Prat Neurol. 2023;14(4):225-36.

20. Bokka KR, Hora S, Jain T, Wambugu M. Deep learning for natural language processing. Birmingham: Packt Publishing; 2019.
21. Vaswani A, Shazeer N, Parmar N, Uszkoreit J, Jones L, Gomez AN, et al. Attention is all you need. Adv Neural Inf Process Syst. 2017;30:1-11.
22. He K, Gan C, Li Z, Rekik I, Yin Z, Ji W, et al. Transformers in medical image analysis. Intell Med. 2023;3(1):59-78.
23. Chu Y, Zhang Y, Wang Q, Zhang L, Wang X, Wang Y, et al. A transformer-based model to predict peptide-HLA class I binding and optimize mutated peptides for vaccine design. Nat Mach Intell. 2022;4(3):300-11.
24. Staudemeyer RC, Morris ER. Understanding LSTM -- a tutorial into long short-term memory recurrent neural networks [Preprint]. ArXiv: 2019. Doi:10.48550/arXiv.1909.09586
25. Levasseur Y. Artificial intelligence techniques for the classification of biological objects in two-dimensional images [ Master's thesis in Engineering]. Quebec City: Université de Québec; 2008.
26. Liang J. Confusion matrix: Machine learning. POGIL Act Clgh. 2022;3(4):1-6.
27. Zemouri R, Devalland C, Valmary-Degano S, Zerhouni N. Artificial intelligence: what future in pathological anatomy? Ann Pathol. 2019;39(2):119-29.
28. Dai Y, Gao Y, Liu F. TransMed: Transformers advance multi-modal medical image classification. Diagnostics. 2021;11(8):1-15.
29. Joumaa H, Sigogne R, Maravic M, Perray L, Bourdin A, Roche N. Artificial intelligence to differentiate asthma from COPD in medico-administrative databases. BMC Pulm Med. 2022;22(1):1-9.

30. Fahrmeir L, Kneib T, Lang S, Marx B. Regression: Models, methods and applications. Berlin, Heidelberg: Springer; 2013.
31. Cornillon PA, Matzner-Løber É. Simple linear regression. In: Cornillon PA, Matzner-Løber É, editors. Regression: Theory and Applications. Paris: Springer; 2007. p. 1-32.
32. Lajugie R. From linear regression to artificial intelligence [Online]. 2019 [Accessed 02/27/2024]. Available from: https://remi-lajugie.fr/docs/regression.pdf
33. Hicham. Formulation and performance of simple and multiple linear regression [Online]. 2022 [Accessed 02/27/2024]. Available at: https://cours-maths-python.com/formulation-performances-regression-lineaire-simple-multiple/
34. Marzell T. Clustering mit Machine Learning - Ein ausführlicher Leitfaden [Online]. 2021 [Accessed on 19/05/2024]. Available at: https://rocketloop.de/de/blog/clustering-machine-learning-ausfuhrlicher-leitfaden/
35. Karim MR, Beyan O, Zappa A, Costa IG, Rebholz-Schuhmann D, Cochez M, et al. Deep learning-based clustering approaches for bioinformatics. Brief Bioinform. 2021;22(1):393-415.
36. Ramesh KK, Kumar GK, Swapna K, Datta D, Rajest SS. A review of medical image segmentation algorithms. Health Technol. 2021;7(27):1-9.
37. Ayesha S, Hanif MK, Talib R. Overview and comparative study of dimensionality reduction techniques for high dimensional data. Inf Fusion. 2020;59:44-58.
38. Journaux L. Multispectral analysis of satellite images and multi-table analysis: application to bird population distribution and landscape structure [Thesis]. Bourgogne : Ecole Doctorale Buffon ; 2006.

39. Zimmer M. Developmental reinforcement learning [Thesis]. Lorraine: Université de Lorraine; 2018.
40. Botvinick M, Wang JX, Dabney W, Miller KJ, Kurth-Nelson Z. Deep reinforcement learning and its neuroscientific implications. Neuron. 2020;107(4):603-16.
41. Youcef Z, Couturier P. Distributed learning approach. Application to trajectory control of a hexapod robot. J Eur Sys Automat. 2005;39:1-29.
42. Lauriola I, Lavelli A, Aiolli F. An introduction to deep learning in natural language processing: Models, techniques, and tools. Neurocomputing. 2022;470:443-56.
43. Borrego-Díaz J, Galán-Páez J. Explainable artificial intelligence in data science. Minds Machines. 2022;32(3):485-531.
44. Shouval R, Fein JA, Savani B, Mohty M, Nagler A. Machine learning and artificial intelligence in haematology. Br J Haematol. 2021;192(2):239-50.
45. Acevedo A, Alférez S, Merino A, Puigví L, Rodellar J. Recognition of peripheral blood cell images using convolutional neural networks. Comput Methods Programs Biomed. 2019;180:1-16.
46. Gedefaw L, Liu CF, Ip RK, Tse HF, Yeung MH, Yip SP, et al. Artificial intelligence-assisted diagnostic cytology and genomic testing for hematologic disorders. Cells. 2023;12(13):1-28.
47. Ahmed I, Balestrieri E, Tudosa I, Lamonaca F. Segmentation techniques for morphometric measurements of blood cells: Overview and research challenges. Meas Sens. 2022;24:1-12.
48. Rodellar J, Alférez S, Acevedo A, Molina A, Merino A. Image processing and machine learning in the morphological analysis of blood cells. Int J Lab Hematol. 2018;40(1):46-53.

49. Cella vision proficiency software. Workflow [Online]. 2024 [Accessed 12/03/2024]. Available at: https://cellavision-proficiency.com/workflow/
50. Surcouf C, Delaune D, Samson T, Foissaud V. Image analysis in haematological cytology: CellaVision DM96 TM Automate. Ann Biol Clin. 2009;67(4):419-24.
51. Katz BZ, Feldman MD, Tessema M, Benisty D, Toles GS, Andre A, et al. Evaluation of Scopio Labs X100 Full Field PBS: The first high-resolution full field viewing of peripheral blood specimens combined with artificial intelligence-based morphological analysis. Int J Lab Hematol. 2021;43(6):1408-16.
52. Scopio. See More. Do More. Diagnose Faster [Online]. 2021 [Accessed on 16/04/2024]. Available at: https://scopiolabs.com/peripheral-blood-smear/
53. Bruegel M, George TI, Feng B, Allen TR, Bracco D, Zahniser DJ, et al. Multicenter evaluation of the cobas m 511 integrated hematology analyzer. Int J Lab Hematol. 2018;40(6):672-82.
54. Zini G, Mancini F, Rossi E, Landucci S, d'Onofrio G. Artificial intelligence and the blood film: Performance of the MC-80 digital morphology analyzer in samples with neoplastic and reactive cell types. Int J Lab Hematol. 2023;45(6):881-9.
55. Merino A, Laguna J, Rodríguez-García M, Julian J, Casanova A, Molina A. Performance of the new MC-80 automated digital cell morphology analyser in detection of normal and abnormal blood cells: Comparison with the CellaVision DM9600. Int J Lab Hematol. 2024;46(1):72-82.

56. Bachar N, Benbassat D, Brailovsky D, Eshel Y, Glück D, Levner D, et al. An artificial intelligence-assisted diagnostic platform for rapid near-patient hematology. Am J Hematol. 2021;96(10):1264-74.
57. Bransky A, Larsson A, Aardal E, Ben-Yosef Y, Christenson RH. A novel approach to hematology testing at the point of care. J Appl Lab Med. 2021;6(2):532-42.
58. Dale DC, Kelley ML, Navarro-De La Vega M, Parthasarathy D, Bodapati D, Virey L, et al. A novel device suitable for home monitoring of white blood cell and neutrophil counts. Blood. 2018;132(1):1-4.
59. U.S. Food & Drug Administration. K181288. U.S.A: FDA; 2018.
60. Zhang Q, Zhong K, Zhang X, Hua C, Kong T, Li J, et al. Artificial intelligence-based Morphogo system: Identification of the morphology of bone marrow nucleated cells with high accuracy [Preprint]. Res Square. 2022. DOI: https://doi.org/10.21203/rs.3.rs-1598923/v1
61. Mallesh N, Zhao M, Meintker L, Höllein A, Elsner F, Lüling H, et al. Knowledge transfer to enhance the performance of deep learning models for automated classification of B cell neoplasms. Patterns. 2021;2(10):1-11.
62. Luo S, Shi Y, Chin LK, Hutchinson PE, Zhang Y, Chierchia G, et al. Machine-learning-assisted intelligent imaging flow cytometry: A review. Adv Intell Syst. 2021;3(11):1-21.
63. Zhao M, Mallesh N, Höllein A, Schabath R, Haferlach C, Haferlach T, et al. Hematologist-level classification of mature B-cell neoplasm using deep learning on multiparameter flow cytometry data. Cytometry A. 2020;97(10):1073-80.
64. Ko BS, Wang YF, Li JL, Li CC, Weng PF, Hsu SC, et al. Clinically validated machine learning algorithm for detecting residual diseases

with multicolor flow cytometry analysis in acute myeloid leukemia and myelodysplastic syndrome. EBioMedicine. 2018;37:91-100.

65. Ng DP, Simonson PD, Tarnok A, Lucas F, Kern W, Rolf N, et al. Recommendations for using artificial intelligence in clinical flow cytometry. Cytometry B Clin Cytom [In Press]. doi: 10.1002/cyto.b.22166.
66. Radakovich N, Nagy M, Nazha A. Machine learning in haematological malignancies. Lancet Haematol. 2020;7(7):541-50.
67. Saleh HM, Saad NH, Isa NA. Overlapping chromosome segmentation using U-Net: convolutional networks with test time augmentation. Procedia Comput Sci. 2019;159:524-33.
68. Deulofeu M, Kolářová L, Salvadó V, María Peña-Méndez E, Almáši M, Štork M, et al. Rapid discrimination of multiple myeloma patients by artificial neural networks coupled with mass spectrometry of peripheral blood plasma. Sci Rep. 2019;9(1):1-7.
69. Acosta J, Ssozi D, Van Galen P. Single-Cell RNA sequencing to disentangle the blood system. Arterioscler Thromb Vasc Biol. 2021;41(3):1012-8.
70. Lee SI, Celik S, Logsdon BA, Lundberg SM, Martins TJ, Oehler VG, et al. A machine learning approach to integrate big data for precision medicine in acute myeloid leukemia. Nat Commun. 2018;9(1):1-13.
71. Akter F, Hossin MA, Daiyan GM, Hossain MM. Classification of hematological data using data mining technique to predict diseases. J Comput Commun. 2018;6(4):76-83.
72. Matek C, Schwarz S, Spiekermann K, Marr C. Human-level recognition of blast cells in acute myeloid leukaemia with convolutional neural networks. Nat Mach Intell. 2019;1(11):538-44.

73. Boldú L, Merino A, Alférez S, Molina A, Acevedo A, Rodellar J. Automatic recognition of different types of acute leukaemia in peripheral blood by image analysis. J Clin Pathol. 2019;72(11):755-61.
74. Matek C, Krappe S, Münzenmayer C, Haferlach T, Marr C. Highly accurate differentiation of bone marrow cell morphologies using deep neural networks on a large image data set. Blood. 2021;138(20):1917-27.
75. Achi HE, Belousova T, Chen L, Wahed A, Wang I, Hu Z, et al. Automated diagnosis of lymphoma with digital pathology images using deep learning. Ann Clin Lab Sci. 2019;49(2):153-60.
76. Sahlol AT, Kollmannsberger P, Ewees AA. Efficient classification of white blood cell leukemia with improved swarm optimization of deep features. Sci Rep. 2020;10:1-11.
77. Mohlman JS, Leventhal SD, Hansen T, Kohan J, Pascucci V, Salama ME. Improving augmented human intelligence to distinguish burkitt lymphoma from diffuse large B-cell lymphoma cases. Am J Clin Pathol. 2020;153(6):743-59.
78. Syrykh C, Abreu A, Amara N, Siegfried A, Maisongrosse V, Frenois FX, et al. Accurate diagnosis of lymphoma on whole-slide histopathology images using deep learning. NPJ Digit Med. 2020;3:1-8.
79. Gunčar G, Kukar M, Notar M, Brvar M, Černelč P, Notar M, et al. An application of machine learning to haematological diagnosis. Sci Rep. 2018;8(1):1-12.
80. Im H, Pathania D, McFarland PJ, Sohani AR, Degani I, Allen M, et al. Design and clinical validation of a point-of-care device for the diagnosis of lymphoma via contrast-enhanced microholography and machine learning. Nat Biomed Eng. 2018;2(9):666-74.

81. Moraes LO, Pedreira CE, Barrena S, Lopez A, Orfao A. A decision-tree approach for the differential diagnosis of chronic lymphoid leukemias and peripheral B-cell lymphomas. Comput Methods Programs Biomed. 2019;178:85-90.
82. Radakovich N, Meggendorfer M, Malcovati L, Hilton CB, Sekeres MA, Shreve J, et al. A geno-clinical decision model for the diagnosis of myelodysplastic syndromes. Blood Adv. 2021;5(21):4361-9.
83. Malcovati L, Stevenson K, Papaemmanuil E, Neuberg D, Bejar R, Boultwood J, et al. SF3B1-mutant MDS as a distinct disease subtype: A proposal from the international working group for the prognosis of MDS. Blood. 2020;136(2):157-70.
84. Chandradevan R, Aljudi AA, Drumheller BR, Kunananthaseelan N, Amgad M, Gutman DA, et al. Machine-based detection and classification for bone marrow aspirate differential counts: initial development focusing on nonneoplastic cells. Lab Invcst. 2020;100(1):98-109.
85. Alaggio R, Amador C, Anagnostopoulos I, Attygalle AD, Araujo IB, Berti E, et al. The 5th edition of the world health organization classification of haematolymphoid tumours: Lymphoid neoplasms. Leukemia. 2022;36(7):1720-48.
86. Walter W, Pohlkamp C, Meggendorfer M, Nadarajah N, Kern W, Haferlach C, et al. Artificial intelligence in hematological diagnostics: Game changer or gadget? Blood Rev. 2023;58:1-11.
87. Chulián S, Martínez-Rubio Á, Pérez-García VM, Rosa M, Blázquez Goñi C, Rodríguez Gutiérrez JF, et al. High-dimensional analysis of single-cell flow cytometry data predicts relapse in childhood acute lymphoblastic leukaemia. Cancers. 2020;13(1):1-20.

88. Shouval R, Labopin M, Bondi O, Mishan-Shamay H, Shimoni A, Ciceri F, et al. Prediction of allogeneic hematopoietic stem-cell transplantation mortality 100 days after transplantation using a machine learning algorithm: A European group for blood and marrow transplantation acute leukemia working party retrospective data mining study. J Clin Oncol. 2015;33(28):3144-51.
89. Ryan L, Mataraso S, Siefkas A, Pellegrini E, Barnes G, Green-Saxena A, et al. A machine learning approach to predict deep venous thrombosis among hospitalized patients. Clin Appl Thromb. 2021;27:1-7.
90. Guglielmelli P, Lasho TL, Rotunno G, Mudireddy M, Mannarelli C, Nicolosi M, et al. MIPSS70: Mutation-enhanced international prognostic score system for transplant-age patients with primary myelofibrosis. J Clin Oncol. 2018;36(4):310-8.
91. MIPSS70 score. MIPSS70-plus version 2.0 score [Online]. 2018 [Accessed 04/17/2024]. Available from: http://www.mipss70score.it/
92. Gresele P. Artificial intelligence and machine learning in hemostasis and thrombosis. Bleeding Thromb Vasc Biol. 2023;2(4):1-6.
93. Nafee T, Gibson CM, Travis R, Yee MK, Kerneis M, Chi G, et al. Machine learning to predict venous thrombosis in acutely ill medical patients. Res Pract Thromb Haemost. 2020;4(2):230-7.
94. Cohen AT, Harrington R, Goldhaber SZ, Hull R, Gibson CM, Hernandez AF, et al. The design and rationale for the acute medically Ill venous thromboembolism prevention with extended duration betrixaban (APEX) study. Am Heart J. 2014;167(3):335-41.
95. Wang HX, Han B, Zhao YY, Kou L, Guo LL, Sun TW, et al. Serum D-dimer as a potential new biomarker for prognosis in patients with thrombotic thrombocytopenic purpura. Medicine. 2020;99(13):1-7.

96. Rashidi HH, Bowers KA, Reyes Gil M. Machine learning in the coagulation and hemostasis arena: An overview and evaluation of methods, review of literature, and future directions. J Thromb Haemost. 2023;21(4):728-43.
97. Rawat J, Virmani J, Singh A, Bhadauria HS, Kumar I, Devgan JS. FAB classification of acute leukemia using an ensemble of neural networks. Evol Intell. 2022;15(1):99-117.
98. Shafique S, Tehsin S. Acute lymphoblastic leukemia detection and classification of its subtypes using pretrained deep convolutional neural networks. Technol Cancer Res Treat. 2018;17:1-7.
99. Rehman A, Abbas N, Saba T, Rahman SI, Mehmood Z, Kolivand H. Classification of acute lymphoblastic leukemia using deep learning. Microsc Res Tech. 2018;81(11):1310-7.
100. Herishanu S. AI-based clinical decision support system for treatment of chronic lymphocytic leukemia/small lymphocytic lymphoma (CLL/SLL) and prediction of treatment efficiency. Blood. 2022;140(1):12393-4.
101. Rashidi HH, Tran N, Albahra S, Dang LT. Machine learning in health care and laboratory medicine: General overview of supervised learning and Auto-ML. Int J Lab Hematol. 2021;43(1):15-22.
102. Kim G, Jo Y, Cho H, Min HS, Park Y. Learning-based screening of hematologic disorders using quantitative phase imaging of individual red blood cells. Biosens Bioelectron. 2019;123:69-76.
103. Jonsson A. Deep reinforcement learning in medicine. Kidney Dis. 2018;5(1):18-22.
104. Alizadeh AA, Eisen MB, Davis RE, Ma C, Lossos IS, Rosenwald A, et al. Distinct types of diffuse large B-cell lymphoma identified by gene expression profiling. Nature. 2000;403:503-11.

105. Prelaj A, Miskovic V, Zanitti M, Trovo F, Genova C, Viscardi G, et al. Artificial intelligence for predictive biomarker discovery in immuno-oncology: A systematic review. Ann Oncol. 2024;35(1):29-65.

106. Gutton J, Lin F, Billuart O, Lajonchère JP, Crubilié C, Sauvage C, et al. L'intelligence artificielle au service des départements d'information médicale: Construction et évaluation d'un outil d'aide à la décision pour cibler et prioriser les séjours à contrôler et fiabiliser les recettes hospitalières générées par la tarification à l'activité. Rev Epidemiol Sante Publique. 2022;70(1):1-8.

107. Doctoroff L, Herzig SJ. Predicting patients at risk for prolonged hospital stays. Med Care. 2020;58(9):778-84.

108. Hub Institute. The future of healthcare with AI for patient management [Online]. 2024 [Accessed 05/21/2024]. Available at: https://www.hubinstitute.com/articles/le-futur-de-la-sante-lia-au-service-de-la-gestion-des-patients

109. Mao AX, Thakkar I. Lost in translation: the vital role of medical translation in global medical communication. Am Med Writ Assoc J. 2023;38(3):4-7.

110. Allegra A, Tonacci A, Sciaccotta R, Genovese S, Musolino C, Pioggia G, et al. Machine learning and deep learning applications in multiple myeloma diagnosis, prognosis, and treatment selection. Cancers. 2022;14(3):1-16.

111. Shreve JT, Khanani SA, Haddad TC. Artificial Intelligence in Oncology: Current Capabilities, Future Opportunities, and Ethical Considerations. Am Soc Clin Oncol Educ Book. 2022 Apr;42:1-10.

112. Allam M, Cai S, Coskun AF. Multiplex bioimaging of single-cell spatial profiles for precision cancer diagnostics and therapeutics. NPJ Precis Oncol. 2020;4:1-14.

113. Lozada JR, Ali A, Day A, Myers JA, Boytim E, Bergom H, et al. A pan-cancer single-cell transcriptomic atlas of natural killer (NK) cells reveals intrinsic and extrinsic mediators of NK cell anti-tumor functions. Blood. 2023;142:2547.
114. Nazha A, Sekeres MA, Bejar R, Rauh MJ, Othus M, Komrokji RS, et al. Genomic biomarkers to predict resistance to hypomethylating agents in patients with myelodysplastic syndromes using artificial intelligence. JCO Precis Oncol. 2019;3:1-11.
115. Boldú L, Merino A, Acevedo A, Molina A, Rodellar J. A deep learning model (ALNet) for the diagnosis of acute leukaemia lineage using peripheral blood cell images. Comput Methods Programs Biomed. 2021;202:1-13.
116. Lipes A, Milena A. Deep learning system for the automatic classification of normal and dysplastic peripheral blood cells as a support tool for the diagnosis [Thesis]. Barcelona: Faculty of Medicine and Health Sciences; 2021.
117. Ingber DE. Is it time for reviewer 3 to request human organ chip experiments instead of animal validation studies? Adv Sci. 2020;7(22):1-15.
118. Arizkane K, Geistlich K, Moindrot L, Risson E, Jeanpierre S, Barral L, et al. A human bone marrow 3D model to investigate the dynamics and interactions between resident cells in physiological or tumoral contexts. J Vis Exp. 2022;190:1-14.
119. Hermange G, Cournède PH, Plo I. Mathematical modeling of hematopoiesis and hematopathies: Development, dynamics and treatment. Hematology. 2022;28(4):183-200.

120. Matteini F, Mulaw MA, Florian MC. Aging of the hematopoietic stem cell niche: New tools to answer an old question. Front Immunol. 2021;12:1-21.
121. Yang F, Poostchi M, Yu H, Zhou Z, Silamut K, Yu J, et al. Deep learning for smartphone-based malaria parasite detection in thick blood smears. IEEE J Biomed Health Inform. 2022;24(5):1427-38.
122. Ghermi M, Messedi M, Berrazeg ZI, Djazouli MA, Ghoumari N, Mened N, et al. Development of artificial intelligence algorithms for immunohematological diagnosis of active tuberculosis. Rev Mal Respir Actual. 2024;16(1):9.
123. De Saint-Affrique D. Artificial intelligence and medicine: What ethical and legal rules for responsible AI? Med Droit. 2022;2022(172):5-7.
124. Qian J, Song T, Zhang Q, Cai G, Cai M. Analysis and diagnosis of hemolytic specimens by AU5800 biochemical analyzer combined with AI technology. Front Comput Intell Sys. 2024;6(3):100-3.
125. Rizzuto V, Mencattini A, Álvarez-González B, Di Giuseppe D, Martinelli E, Beneitez-Pastor D, et al. Combining microfluidics with machine learning algorithms for RBC classification in rare hereditary hemolytic anemia. Sci Rep. 2021;11(1):1-12.
126. Mallappallil M, Sabu J, Gruessner A, Salifu M. A review of big data and medical research. SAGE Open Med. 2020;8:1-10.
127. Moingeon P, Garbay C, Dahan M, Fermont I, Benmakhlouf A, Gouyette A, et al. Artificial intelligence, a revolution in drug development. Med Sci. 2024;40(4):369-76.
128. Moingeon P, Kuenemann M, Guedj M. Artificial intelligence-enhanced drug design and development: Toward a computational precision medicine. Drug Discov Today. 2022;27(1):215-22.

129. Miotto R, Wang F, Wang S, Jiang X, Dudley JT. Deep learning for healthcare: Review, opportunities and challenges. Brief Bioinform. 2018;19(6):1236-46.
130. Gedefaw L, Liu CF, Ip RK, Tse HF, Yeung MH, Yip SP, et al. Artificial intelligence-assisted diagnostic cytology and genomic testing for hematologic disorders. Cells. 2023;12(13):1-28.
131. Zech JR, Badgeley MA, Liu M, Costa AB, Titano JJ, Oermann EK. Variable generalization performance of a deep learning model to detect pneumonia in chest radiographs: A cross-sectional study. PLoS Med. 2018;15(11):e1002683.
132. Schmidt C. M. D. Anderson breaks with IBM watson, raising questions about artificial intelligence in oncology. J Natl Cancer Inst. 2017;109(5):4-5.
133. Commission nationale de l'informatique et des libertés. How can we keep the human touch? Report on the ethical challenges of algorithms and artificial intelligence. Paris: CNIL; 2017.
134. World Health Organization. WHO issues first global report on Artificial Intelligence (AI) in health and six guiding principles for its design and use. Geneva: WHO; 2021.
135. European Union. Regulation (EU) 2021/821 of the European Parliament and of the Council of 20 May 2021. Official Journal of June 11, 2021.
136. Data-driven control and AI in healthcare: bringing the "Human Guarantee" MedTech and HealthTech ecosystem to life! Ann Mines. 2022;3:24-6.

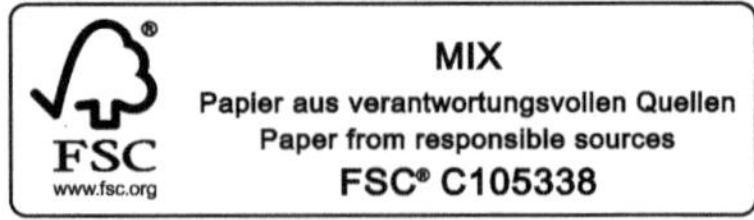


Printed by Books on Demand GmbH, Norderstedt / Germany